PET-CT in Infection and Inflammation

Sikandar Shaikh

PET-CT in Infection and Inflammation

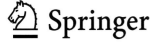 Springer

Dr. Sikandar Shaikh
Consultant PET-CT & Radiology
Yashoda Hospitals
Somajiguda, Hyderabad
Telangana
India

Assistant Professor, Department of Radiodiagnosis
Shadan Institute of Medical Sciences
Hyderabad
Telangana
India

Adjunct Assistant Professor, Department of Biomedical Engineering
Indian Institute of Technology
Hyderabad
Telangana
India

ISBN 978-981-15-9800-5   ISBN 978-981-15-9801-2   (eBook)
https://doi.org/10.1007/978-981-15-9801-2

This Springer imprint is published by the registered company Springer Nature Singapore Pte Ltd.
The registered company address is: 152 Beach Road, #21-01/04 Gateway East, Singapore 189721,
Singapore

This book is dedicated to

*Almighty God whose blessings are
always there*

*My parents whatever today i am is because
of them*

*My wife continous source of encouragement
and motivation*

My daughters

*My mentors who made me to do best
everytime*

My teachers who taught me everything

My well-wishers

*My friends, my colleagues and my entire
department staff of Radiology, PET-CT and
Nuclear Medicine for their valuable support*

*My patients because of whom I learnt the art
of medicine and Radiology and still learning*

Foreword

It is my great pleasure to write a foreword for this book that has been written by Dr. Sikandar Shaikh. PET-CT scan has revolutionized the discipline of medical imaging during the last two decades. This innovation has led to enhancing the concept of personalized medicine for effective medical care for patients with serious diseases and disorders. With further advances made using this technology and the introduction of novel radiotracers in recent years, PET imaging has become an essential necessity in the day-to-day practice of medicine. While applications of PET have mostly dealt with managing patients with cancer and neurological disorders, its role in other domains has been increasingly explored in recent years. Infection and inflammation are the most common sources of morbidity and mortality worldwide but are suboptimally managed with the existing techniques. PET-CT is a powerful molecular imaging modality which has proven to be the most sensitive and specific imaging methodology in assessing many disease processes. With the advances made it is feasible to screen the entire body within a short period of time non-invasively and quantify the underlying process with high precision and accuracy. In this comprehensive book about the impact of PET-CT imaging in assessing infection and inflammation, Dr. Sikandar Shaikh describes the importance and the critical role of FDG-PET/CT in this quite common entity in medicine. By now it is well established that inflammatory cells are highly glycolytic, and therefore, sites of infection and inflammation can be detected and localized by this imaging technique. Currently, FDG is the tracer of choice for this purpose, but this potential is being explored by testing other compounds. In this book, applications of FDG-PET imaging are described in detail in many known infectious and inflammatory entities. Despite advances made by introducing numerous laboratory tests to diagnose such disorders, medical imaging plays an essential role in the management of patients with highly effective therapeutic interventions. PET-CT imaging allows localizing and quantifying disease activity at various stages of the disease and guiding invasive intervention if clinically indicated.

I have known Dr. Sikandar Shaikh as a distinguished colleague and an academician par excellence in our discipline. He has been involved as a major contributor to many international organizations. He is President Elect of ISMRM India Chapter, Indian Ambassador of the European Society of Hybrid, Molecular and Translational Imaging, Education Committee Member of the World Molecular Imaging Society, Oncoimaging Committee Society for Pediatric Radiology, Education Committee ISMRM

International, Research Committee European Society of Oncoimaging, and various National Indian Radiological Sub Societies. He is reviewer of *AJR*, *BJR*, *European Radiology*, *JMRI*, *Radiology*, *Radiographics*, *Radiology: Cardiothoracic Imaging*, and many more journals. He has made many presentations in various International and national societies. Therefore, I believe, this book will be a great source of information on this topic for the clinicians, radiologists, nuclear physicians, and residents from various specialities. With this introduction I wish him all the best for publishing this book and all his future endeavors.

Philadelphia, PA   Abas Alavi, MD, MD(Hon), PhD(Hon), DSc(Hon)
26th July 2020   University of Pennsylvania
                                                                        Philadelphia, PA
                                                                                    USA

Foreword

On the Editor

Dr. Sikandar Shaikh, DMRD, DNB, MNAMS, FICR, is Consultant PET-CT and Radiology at Yashoda Hospitals in Hyderabad; Assistant Professor at Shadan Medical College, Hyderabad; and Adjunct Assistant Professor at the Department of Biomedical Engineering in Hyderabad, India. He is President Elect of the ISMRM India Chapter and CCM Member of the Telangana State Chapter of IRIA. Dr. Sikandar takes responsibility as the Ambassador of the European Society of Hybrid and Translational Imaging (ESHI) in India, as a Research committee member of the European Society of Oncological Imaging (ESOI), as an Education committee member of the World Molecular Imaging Society (WMIS), as a member of the Oncoimaging committee in the International Society of Pediatric Radiology (SPR), and as Governing Council Member of the Society of Emergency Radiology (SER) India. Dr. Sikandar is author or co-author of multiple International publications and serves as Associate editor of the *Journal of Magnetic Resonance Imaging* (JMRI).

Foreword PET/CT in Infection and Inflammation

Infectious diseases represent a major cause of mortality, and chronic inflammation has been identified as the cause of many systemic disorders with a wide spectrum of immune-related clinical manifestations. The discovery of new infectious agents and a progressing understanding of the complex immune response to intrinsic and extrinsic stimuli have markedly altered traditional concepts of inflammation. The causal role of infectious agents in chronic inflammatory disease and cancer has major implications for public health, treatment, and prevention. Imaging is a pillar of diagnostic and therapeutic management in patients with inflammatory disease: localization of the primary inflammatory focus and secondary manifestations, longitudinal therapy monitoring, and complication management and interventional procedure planning are directly guiding therapeutic strategy.

Most relevant imaging modalities for local and whole-body imaging of inflammation and infection include computed tomography (CT), magnetic resonance imaging (MRI), ultrasound, and hybrid imaging techniques (PET/CT, PET/MRI,

SPECT). At the beginning of the diagnostic algorithm stands the search for a possible primary inflammatory focus. Clinically, conventional whole-body contrast-enhanced CT is most frequently used as first line. Beyond morphology, multiple studies indicate augmented diagnostic accuracy of PET/CT with ^{18}F-fluorodeoxyglucose (^{18}F-FDG) for the detection of an infectious focus and longitudinal assessment of inflammatory activity by the complementary integration of glucose metabolism into the diagnostic algorithm. ^{18}F-FDG PET/CT has demonstrated additional diagnostic value in a broad spectrum of inflammatory disease, ranging from fever of unknown origin, tuberculosis and HIV, prosthesis infections in orthopedics, and vascular grafts to aseptic autoimmune disease with manifestations such as vasculitis, arteriosclerosis, arthritis, and graft-versus-host disease. Beyond FDG with significant advances in the understanding of immunologic response in inflammation and cancer, immuno-PET targeting specific innate immune mediators is under development in mostly experimental settings to characterize the pathophysiology of inflammation in greater detail than ever. Increasing evidence advocates that multiparametric molecular imaging of inflammatory response contributes significantly to the individualized management of infectious and inflammatory disease with a substantial impact on value-based therapeutic strategy and health outcome for the patient. In perspective, comprehensive pathophysiological characterization of infectious and inflammatory diseases necessitates the multiparametric integration of imaging and tissue-based and laboratory parameters to provide diagnostic biomarkers to guide therapeutic strategy with a beneficial impact on the efficiency of treatment and patient outcome.

Clemens Cyran
President ESHI European Society of Hybrid
Molecular and Translational Imaging
Section Chief Hybrid and Molecular Imaging
Department of Radiology
Munich, Germany   Ludwig-Maximillian's-University Munich
26th July 2020   Munich, Germany

Foreword

I have great pleasure in writing a foreword for this book. PET-CT scan is in use for the last few years. Initially, it was popular in detecting and studying cancer. It is also used for following up during and after the treatment of cancer. Dr. Sikandar Shaikh also brings out the importance of use of PET-CT scan in Infection and Inflammations. F-FDG PET/CT is being widely used for imaging of infectious and inflammatory diseases. It has been demonstrated that cells involved in infection and inflammation, especially neutrophils and the monocyte/macrophage family, are able to express high levels of glucose transporters and hexokinase activity. PET scan reveals the functional and metabolic activities, while CT scan outlines the anatomical area. PET-CT using FDG has many advantages which are revealed in this book. The basic physics and techniques are also mentioned. The inflammations and infections involving the various body organ systems and their identification are described and illustrated in this book. Despite the wide use of antibiotics and anti-inflammatory drugs, these are still rampant contributing to morbidity and mortality.

I know Dr. Sikandar Shaikh for the last two decades and found out that he is a dynamic, hardworking, and dedicated radiologist. Apart from his organizational ability, his teaching and academic activities have been appreciated by many. I am sure that this book will become popular and encourage him to write some more on specified topics. I wish him all the best in his efforts.

Kakarla Subbarao, MBBS, MS, FACR, FRCR, DSC (Hon)
Nizam's Institute of Medical Sciences, KREST

Hyderabad, India
26th July 2020

Hyderabad, Telangana
India

Foreword

I am pleased to write this foreword, not only because of Dr. Sikandar being a good friend for more than 20 years, and a renowned PET-CT and Radiology consultant, but also because I strongly believe in the educative value this book offers in the field of radiology. It offers detailed information about PET-CT in Infection and inflammation and aims to benefit the larger medical community.

Dr. Sikandar has always been keen on the concept of Infection and inflammation. I recall we would carry out discussions when we worked together at Yavatmal Medical College, in the rural area of Vidarbha region in Maharashtra State, India, with hardly any investigation facilities and hundreds of patients. He was instrumental in setting up CT scan machine and helping the clinicians single-handedly and working relentlessly in this medical college. I hope he will not forget sitting in the only Internet cafe in Yavatmal, where he pursued new learning and researches in the field of radiology.

Over a long and fruitful career, Dr. Sikandar has worked in four hospitals across India and has published in various journals. A lot of important book chapters grew out of his work and experience in PET-CT scanning. He has also presented his papers numerous times internationally and received many awards and recognitions throughout his career.

Being an ardent researcher and a scholar, Dr. Sikandar has produced a powerful tool for thoughtful and sustained practice in radiology. Through this book, he presents to you the abstract version of his intellectual foundations in PET-CT. I hope this book will become a textbook for those wanting to excel by drawing a correlation between PET-CT and infectious diseases.

Happy Reading

Nagpur, India   Major Milind Bhuchandi, MD
26th July 2020

Preface

The use of PET-CT in imaging had a major impact on assessing the various diseases and pathologies. After the introduction of PET-CT, FDG-PET-CT scanning has become a more powerful imaging modality. Its superiority over routinely used conventional imaging modalities such as computed tomography (CT) and magnetic resonance imaging in the characterization and evaluation of the lesion with high sensitivity and specificity has made it the most preferred imaging modality.

PET-CT in infection and inflammation is a new concept in imaging which has been established in recent days. This is an especially important application which has evolved in recent days. Initially, PET-CT was used only in oncology, but now it is more commonly being used for many benign applications, the majority of it comprising infection and inflammation. The various etiological factors for infection are many like bacterial, viral, parasitic, and fungal causes. The concept of fever of unknown origin is also included in this category of evaluation. This newer application is significantly used so that ideally it becomes possible to evaluate the whole body and make a diagnosis. One of the hallmarks is the Dual point time imaging. This is a delayed PET imaging technique which differentiates between benign and malignant pathologies easily.

This book is written to stress on the various applications related to infection and inflammations which will be used for easier and earlier diagnosis. The message in this book is also to focus on the correct protocols which can be used for better and precise evaluation of the various infective and inflammatory conditions.

Hyderabad, India   Sikandar Shaikh

Acknowledgments

Dr. Abas Alavi, MD, MD(Hon), Ph.D(Hon), DSc (Hon)
Professor of Radiology, University of Pennsylvania, USA.

Prof. Clemens Cyran, MD
President ESHI European Society of Hybrid Molecular and Translational Imaging, Professor of Radiology, Section Chief Hybrid and Molecular Imaging and Vice Chair at the Department of Radiology, Ludwig-Maximillian's-University Munich, Germany

Prof. Kakarla Subbarao, M.B.B.S, MS, FACR, FRCR, DSC (Hon)
Emeritus Professor of Radiology, Nizam's Institute of Medical Sciences, Hyderabad, India. Past President National IRIA.

Dr. Prabhakar Reddy, MD, DMRD
Dean, Professor and Head Department of Radiology, Mahavir Institute of Medical Sciences, Vikarabad. Telangana, India, Past President AOCR and National IRIA

Dr. Anand Abkari, MD(RD), DMR, FICR, FIAMS
Professor Emeritus, Department of Radiology, Deccan College of Medical Sciences, Hyderabad, India

Prof. T. Mandapal, MD, FICR
Director Radiology Services and Head Department of Radiology, CARE Group of Hospitals, Hyderabad, India

Prof. Rammurthi S., MD, MAMS, FICR
Senior, Professor & Head Department of Radiology and Imaging, Dean of Faculty Nizams Institute of Medical Sciences, Hyderabad, India

Dr. Hemant Patel, MD, DNB, DMRE
Director, Gujarat Imaging Centre, Postgraduate Institute of Radiology, Ahmedabad, India. Immediate Past President National IRIA.

Dr. Hrushikesh Aurangabadkar, DNB, DRM
Consultant and Head Department of Nuclear Medicine and PET-CT, Yashoda Hospitals, Somajiguda, Hyderabad, India

Dr. N. Chidambaranathan, MD, DNB, FICR, PhD
Head Department of Radiology,
Apollo Hospitals, Greams Road, Chennai, India

Dr. Arvind Chaturvedi, MD
Prof. and Head Department of Radiology, Rajiv Gandhi Cancer Institute, New Delhi, India
Dr. Milind Bhrushundi, Ex Major AMC
Director Central India Institute of Infectious Diseases and Research (CIIID & R), Medical Director and chief HIV Unit Lata Mangeshkar Hospital, Nagpur, India
Prof. C. Amarnath, MD, DNB, FICR, FRCR, MBA
Professor & HOD, Stanley Medical College, Chennai, India, President Elect National IRIA
Dr. Suresh Kawathekar, MD, DMRD
Professor & HOD Department of Radiology, MNR Medical College, Sanga Reddy, Hyderabad, India
Doguparthi Suresh
Assistant Manager, Yashoda Hospitals, Somajiguda, Hyderabad, India

List of Abbreviations

^{11}C	11 Carbon
^{13}N	13 Nitrogen
^{15}O	15 Oxygen
18F FDG	18 Flourinated fluorodeoxyglucose
18F NaF	18 Sodium fluoride
18F	18 Fluorine
82-Rb	82-Rubidium
99mTC	99 m Technetium
99Tc Bone scan	99 Technetium bone scan
ACR	American College of Radiology
AIDS	Acquired immunodeficiency syndrome
ALARA	As Low as Reasonably Achievable
APD	Avalanche photodiode
ARDS	Adult respiratory distress syndrome
ATP	Adenosine triphosphate
ATT	Anti-tubercular treatment
CD4	Cluster of differentiation 4
CIAP	Clinical inhibitor apoptosis
CKD	Chronic kidney disease
CNS	Central nervous system
COPD	Chronic obstructive pulmonary disease
COVID-19	Coronavirus disease 2019
COVID	Coronavirus disease
CRP	C-reactive protein
CTA	Computed tomography angiogram
DNA	Deoxyribonucleic acid
DOTANOC	DOTA–sodium iodide–octreotide
DPS	Dual point scan
DPTI	Dual point time imaging
DTP	Diphtheria tetanus pertussis
DVT	Deep vein thrombosis
EANM	European Association of Nuclear Medicine
EEG	Electroencephalogram
ESR	Erythrocyte sedimentation rate

EULAR	European League Against Rheumatism
FDG	Fluorodeoxyglucose
FIAU PET	1-(2'-Deoxy-deoxy-2'-fluoro-beta-D-arabinofuranosyl)-5-iodouracil positron emission tomography
FUO	Fever of unknown origin
Ga67-Citrate	Gallium 67 citrate
Ga-68	Gallium 68
GCA	Giant cell arteritis
GI Tract	Gastrointestinal tract
GLUT	Glucose transporter
HAART	Highly active antiretroviral therapy
HCC	Hepatocellular carcinoma
HIV	Human immunodeficiency virus
HU	Hounsfield unit
IBD	Inflammatory bowel disease
ICM Criteria PJI	International Consensus Meeting Criteria Prosthetic Joint Infection
IDSA Criteria PJI	Infectious Diseases Society of America Criteria Prosthetic Joint Infection
IL	Interleukin
IV	Intravenous
KEV	Kiloelectron volt
LAD	Left anterior descending artery
LCA	Left circumflex artery
LCH	Langerhans cell histiocytosis
LCV	Large cell vasculitis
LM	Left main Coronary artery
LSO	Lutetium-oxyorthosilicate
LVAD	Left ventricular assisted device
MDR TB	Multidrug resistant tuberculosis
Mg/dl	Milligram/deciliter
MRI	Magnetic resonance imaging
MSIS Criteria PJI	Musculoskeletal Infection Society Criteria Prosthetic Joint Infection
MTB	Mycobacterium tuberculosis
NET	Neuroendocrine tumor
NPG	Negative predictive value
NSAID'S	Nonsteroidal anti-inflammatory drugs
PCR	Polymerase chain reaction
PE	Pulmonary embolism
PET-MRI	Positron emission tomography magnetic resonance imaging
PET	Positron emission tomography
PET-CT	Positron emission tomography and computed tomography
PJI	Prosthetic joint infection
PMN	Polymorphonuclear neutrophil percentage

PMR	Polymyalgia rheumatica
PMT	Photomultiplier tube
PPV	Positive predictive value
PSMA	Prostate-specific membrane antigen
PTLD	Post-transplant lymphoproliferative disorder
PUO	Pyrexia of unknown origin
RCC	Renal cell carcinoma
RNA	Ribonucleic acid
ROI	Region of interest
RPF	Retroperitoneal fibrosis
SARS	Severe acute respiratory syndrome
SiPM	Silicon photomultiplier
SNM	Society of Nuclear Medicine and Molecular imaging
SPECT	Single-photon emission computed tomography
SPIO	Superparamagnetic iron oxide
SPN	Solitary pulmonary nodule
SSPE	Subacute sclerosing panencephalitis
SUV max	Standardized uptake value maximum
SUV maxd	Standardized uptake value maximum delayed
SUV maxe	Standardized uptake value maximum early
SUV mean	Standardized uptake value mean
SUV	Standardized uptake value
SUV1	Standardized uptake value delayed imaging 1
SUV2	Standardized uptake value delayed imaging 2
SUV3	Standardized uptake value delayed imaging 3
SUV4	Standardized uptake value delayed imaging 4
T-cell	T-Lymphocyte
TOF	Time of flight
TSPO	Translocator protein
USPIO	Ultra-superparamagnetic iron oxide
WBC	White blood cells

Contents

About the Author

Sikandar Shaikh, DMRD, DNB, EDiR, MNAMS, FICR is European Board Certified Radiologist. He is working as a Consultant PET-CT and Radiology at Yashoda Hospitals, Hyderabad, India. He has several peer-reviewed publications and delivered numerous lectures and oral and poster presentations in various International, National, State, regional, and university level meetings. Dr. Shaikh is the elected Secretary of the Indian College of Radiology 2021–2023, President Elect of ISMRM India Chapter, Indian Ambassador of the European Society of Hybrid, Molecular and Translational Imaging (ESHI), Research Committee Member of the European Society of Oncoimaging (ESOI), Education Committee Member of the World Molecular Imaging Society (WMIS) and ISMRM International, Oncoimaging Committee International Society for Pediatric Radiology (SPR), Governing Council Member—Society of Emergency Radiology (SER) India, Ethics Committee Member—IIT Hyderabad, Associate Editor—JMRI (*International Journal of MRI*), and CCM Telangana State Chapter IRIA. He is the Secretary elect for Indian College Of Radiology ICRI 2021–2022.

Introduction

This book is important for the basic clinicians, all subspecialties that are involved in the imaging of the infection and inflammation. This book has described in detail various chapters in relation to infection and inflammation. Each chapter of this book includes detailed descriptions of how Positron Emission Tomography and Computed Tomography PET-CT is being used in the evaluation of the specific infective inflammatory diseases. The description and discussion are also meticulously done with relevant images so that the basic concept of using the PET-CT in infection and inflammatory conditions is explained meticulously. Each chapter is described in detail about the various clinical presentations, including key images and their interpretation, techniques, and diagnosis. After reading this book, it allows readers to understand the value of PET/CT for the diagnosis of fever of unknown origin, tuberculosis, cardiac pathologies, chest pathologies, vasculitis, Polymyalgia Rheumatica, pediatric applications, prosthesis joint infections, organ transplantations, viral infections, and molecular imaging in infection and inflammation. Given the scope of this modality, PET-CT gives a comprehensive review of the various applications for various specialties.

© The Author(s), under exclusive license to Springer Nature
Singapore Pte Ltd. 2021
S. Shaikh, *PET-CT in Infection and Inflammation*,
https://doi.org/10.1007/978-981-15-9801-2_1

PET-CT Physics, Instrumentation, and Techniques

2

2.1 Introduction

The PET-CT is an important imaging modality of molecular imaging. The molecular imaging is defined as the visualization, characterization, and measurement of biological processes at the molecular and cellular levels by the SNM, i.e., Society of Nuclear Medicine and Molecular Imaging [1]. This PET-CT is an important component of hybrid imaging which means a combination of functional and structural imaging for quantification [2, 3]. This imaging modality quantification is done based on the amount of radiotracer uptake in a particular tissue over a period of time. Thus, FDG PET-CT has revolutionized modern medicine with the newer concept of personalized medicine. The PET-CT is widely used in various pathologies on oncology, neurology, cardiology, infection inflammation, and various newer miscellaneous applications [4, 5]. Thus, PET-CT has now been established as an important multidisciplinary imaging modality. PET-CT is being used widely for the evaluation of the malignancies especially for diagnosis, staging and restaging, monitoring response to therapy, and for indications like Radiotherapy planning. PET-CT has also become the important modality for imaging in animal models also to study the various disease pathologies, new drug developments, and various treatment strategies [6]. Thus, PET-CT offers a wide range of information to study the biological and biochemical processes.

PET alone as the functional imaging modality is not specific as the exact location of the anatomical structures needs to be defined. For this fusion of PET with CT or MRI is done and PET-CT/PET-MR is formed by the co-registration of the functional and anatomical images. This is called as Hybrid Imaging.

© The Author(s), under exclusive license to Springer Nature
Singapore Pte Ltd. 2021
S. Shaikh, *PET-CT in Infection and Inflammation*,
https://doi.org/10.1007/978-981-15-9801-2_2

2.2   Principle of PET-CT

2.2.1   Annihilations

PET is based on the basic principle of annihilation process in which the photons are released when the radionuclides emit positrons, and they undergo the annihilation with the electrons [7]. The radiotracer injected is analogous to the common biological molecules present in the body like glucose, peptides, and proteins in the body. These released photons are emitting the energies of 511 keV at exactly opposite to each other [8]. This energy is identified by coincidence imaging by the detectors. This is based on the law of the conservation of energy where the 511-keV represents the energy equivalent of the mass of the electron. In this process of the bombardment of the target material with photons which will be accelerated in the cyclotron for the production of the positron-emitting radionuclides. This forms the basis of the radionuclide production [9].

2.2.2   Radiotracer Techniques

In order to detect the gamma rays due to annihilations, scintillation crystals [10] are used to absorb and convert the high energy gamma rays into low energy photons. With the development of the detector technology lot of limitations of PET are not seen now. The commonly used detectors are Lutetium-Oxyorthosilicate LSO which has remarkably high density, high light output, fast decay time, and excellent resolution. In this process photosensor like PMT, APD, or SiPM is used to convert the light signal into the electrical signal [11]. The amount of PET uptake is directly proportional to the amount of glycolysis in the FDG Radiotracer. The positrons emitted from a radionuclide have enough kinetic energy to travel.

Thus, a lot of factors are important in the sequence of technical, patient-related factors then biokinetics of radiotracer distribution. The amount of physiological uptake and the pathological uptakes.

Evolution of PET was documented in 1934 when Irene and Curie proved the formation of radioactive materials, which decayed by emitting the positrons. The first medical Cyclotron was established by Lawrence to produce the Isotopes [12, 13].

The basic component of PET is made up of multiple ring detection systems consisting of Bismuth germinate oxide (DGO) [14] and cesium fluoride. PET instrumentation is developed parallelly along with the development of radiochemistry. Many compounds like ^{15}O, ^{13}N, ^{11}C, and ^{18}F. Thus, dedicated PET-CT was introduced commercially with the evolution of instrumentation and radiochemical diversity.

2.3   PET Physics

2.3.1   Positron Emission

Positron is a positively charged electron with the same mass of an electron. This positron annihilates with electrons to form photons moving in the opposite direction. Now this annihilation process forms the basis of the PET. Positron emission is based on the isobaric decay process, which is also known as Beta plus decay [15]. In this process, the radionuclides are converted into neutron with release of positron. This positron decay results in the conversion of one isotope into another. In this process of annihilation where the energy is emitted in opposite directions at 180° to each other and can be detected by PET detectors. The most commonly used detectors are LSO (Lutetium Oxyortho Silicate). With the advent of detector development, a lot of new techniques are coming. One technique is TOF (Time of Flight) (Diagrams 2.1 and 2.2).

Positron Emission Tomography (PET) Scanner

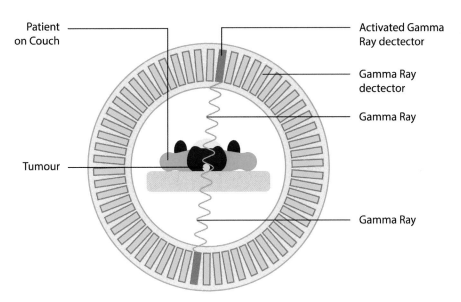

Diagram 2.1 PET-CT gantry showing PET scintillators showing the photon energy being detected at 180° to each other on the basis of the Einstein's principle. This forms the basis of the PET image acquisition

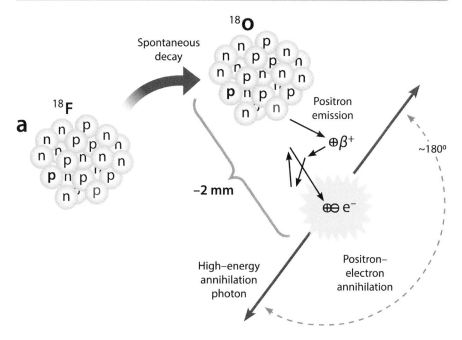

Diagram 2.2 This is the process of positron electron annihilation where the energy released on the basis of the Einstein's principle at 180° to each other which is detected by scintillators

2.3.2 PET Scanner

PET scanners are made up of multiple small detectors that are arranged adjacent to each other and typically the diameter range is from 60 to 90 cm. Around 25,000 detectors are seen in the length of 10–25 cm. PET detectors are high-density scintillator crystals which has a capacity to converts the photon energy. These scintillators are combined to a device known as photomultiplier tube (PMT) [16]. In this process, light is converted into electric signals. These signals from each detector are combined in the coincidence circuit (Diagram 2.3).

2.3.3 PET Image

Thus, PET images are formed by the single voxel images, which are calibrated with the radioactive tracers. Thus, the 511-keV energy from different annihilation processes is clubbed together for the image formation. In this PET-CT, CT has a significant role in attenuation correction. With the advent of technology, a lot of new developments have occurred in PET-CT, one of them is TOF PET.

PET Scanner

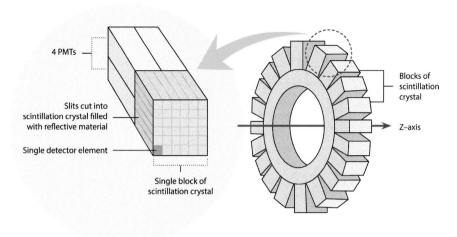

Diagram 2.3 Blocks made up of scintillation crystals with Photomultiplier tubes

2.4   Radiotracers

Many radiotracers are there for the imaging of PET, but the ideal radiotracer depends on the half-life. This half-life for the imaging should be in imaging limits and feasibility, so that it should be injected and transferred in the body and scan should be done in shorter time frames [17]. The shorter half-life of a couple of minutes and a longer half-life in many hours and days are not recommended for imaging. The ideal radiotracer in PET imaging should be comfortable to inject and scan should be done at the same go. These radiotracers are prepared by the synthesis process in Cyclotron [18]. Radiotracer is produced after a couple of reactions. The most commonly used radiotracer is Fluorinateddeoxyglucose (F-FDG). F-18 is being produced in cyclotron by bombarding the O-18 enriched water with high energy protons. Negatively charged hydrogen ions are accelerated in cyclotron forming the positive hydrogen ions that are high energy and directed toward O-18 enriched water. This proton undergoes the nuclear reaction with O-18 forming F-18. The synthesis of the FDG is done from the F-18 component. Thus, the FDG produced is a sterile, pyrogenic, colorless, and clear liquid. This F-FDG is glucose which is tagged with the radioactive material. In this process, the radioactive purity is greater than 95%. The concept of this glucose metabolisms glycolysis which is also known as the Warburg effect [19]. The amount of cellular uptake of FDG is directly proportional to the activity in a particular tissue or an organ. This biochemical process of FDG formation depends on the glucose transporters (GLUT) pathway. Thus, FDG uptake is not only specific for cancer but all other applications like infection and inflammation where there is an increased turnover of the glucose. F-FDG is avid for many pathologies and not sensitive to the diagnosis for all these pathologies. For this many new radiotracers are been invented, which are more organ specific or system specific and can be used easily for the diagnosis. This is becoming the basis of personalized medicine in future (Diagrams 2.4 and 2.5).

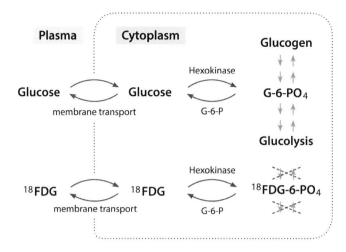

Diagram 2.4 Comparison of the normal glucose and fluorodeoxyglucose metabolism

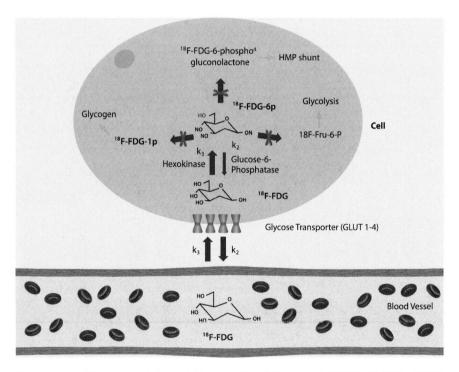

Diagram 2.5 Glucose metabolism within the cell and the role of GLUT1, GLUT2, GLUT3 and GLUT 4

2.5   Factors Influencing FDG Uptake

The malignant cells have important properties of rapid proliferation, increase in size local invasion and distant metastases. The amount of the FDG radiotracer uptake depends on the various factors like the number of tumor cells, grading of tumor, histological subtype, and vascularity. The vascularity of the tumor is related to the amount of oxygen in a particular tissue with less oxygen, this entity is known as tumor hypoxia [20] (Diagrams 2.6 and 2.7).

This is the same principle of the PET in infection and inflammation. Sometimes it becomes difficult to differentiate between different pathologies as many of them will have same amount of uptake. Here some criteria are there to differentiate between them but still a few cases a little difficult. For this, the advancements in the radiotracers are also there where in the future it will be more focused to evaluate pathologies in relation to the radiotracer pathologies (Diagram 2.8).

The amount of FDG uptake in a particular tissue whether physiological or pathological depends on the amount of the uptake, which is quantified by standardized uptake values (SUV) [21].

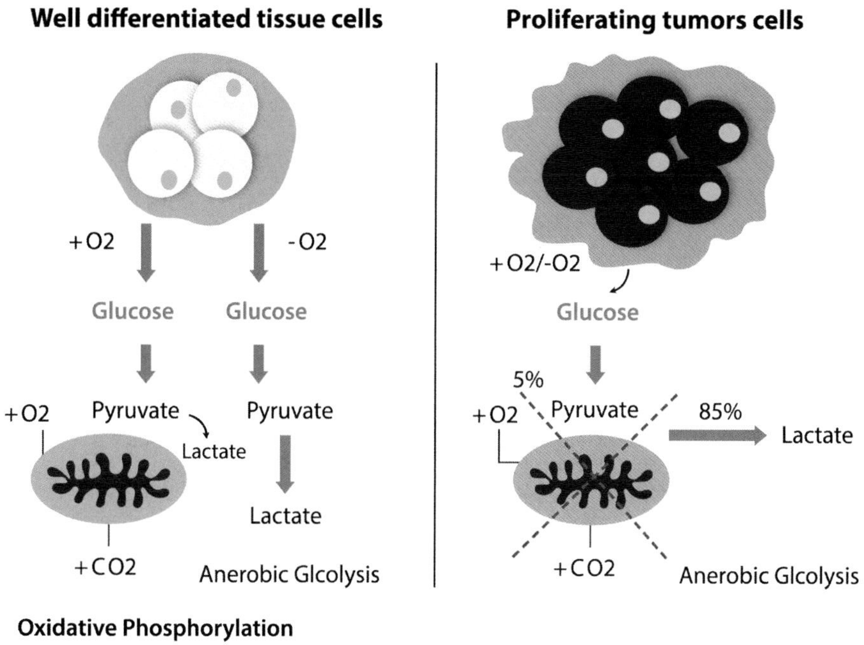

Well differentiated tissue cells   **Proliferating tumors cells**

Oxidative Phosphorylation

Diagram 2.6 Glucose metabolism in normal tissues and tumor tissues. In normal tissues, the oxidative phosphorylation takes place while in tumor proliferating cells it does not take place

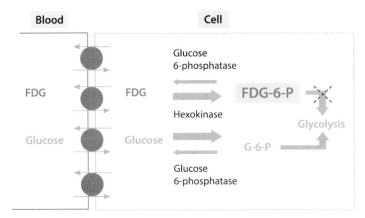

Mechanism of FDG uptake in tumor cell

Diagram 2.7 Metabolism of FDG in tumor cells, the FDG 6 phosphate to glycolysis does not take place

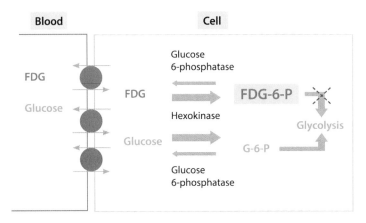

Mechanism of FDG uptake in inflammatory cells

Diagram 2.8 Metabolism of FDG in inflammatory cells. The FDG 6 Phosphate to glycolysis does not take place. Thus, the mechanism of metabolism is same in both the processes

2.6   PET-CT Scanning Technique

2.6.1   Patient Preparation

Fasting for 4–6 h is needed before the PET-CT scan. This is the optimal duration needed for the optimum uptake in pathological tissues. To avoid caffeinated and alcoholic beverages. The amount of uptake depends on glucose metabolism in a particular tissue. It is important to know the knowledge of the distribution, physiologic uptake, and common normal variants [22]. False increased or decreased blood glucose levels needs to be quantified. The ideal blood sugar level should be below 150 mg/dl. The blood sugar levels at higher levels, above 200 mg/dl, should be rescheduled. The blood sugar levels between 150 and 200 mg/dl [23] should be administered insulin to reduce the blood sugar levels. False-positive results can be seen in insulin-induced hypoglycemia. The average dose of FDG uptake is 10 mCi which is injected intravenously. No obvious contraindications for FDG injection are there. Ideally scan is done after 60 min of the FDG injection. The ideal position is arms up position this is needed to reduce the beam hardening artifacts while doing CT. The various protocols of whole-body imaging are there, base of the skull to mid-thigh is the standard and most widely used protocol practiced throughout the world. Limited PET-CT scans are usually done for cardiac, neurological applications, and prosthetic joint infections imaging. Upper and lower limbs scan to be done separately along with the whole-body scan. This again depends on the indications like melanoma or any specific clinical symptoms in the upper or lower limb.

2.6.2   CT Technique

As per the sequence of events in PET-CT, CT is done first followed by PET. Different protocols are being used for CT, that is, plain CT, single phase study, or triphasic study depending on the organs involved [24]. Triphasic CECT is planned in cases of neuroendocrine tumors, hemangioma liver, etc. This planning is an integral part of PET-CT planning. This CT imaging is done in the proper inspiratory phase. Lung window acquisition to be done separately after whole-body scan to delineate the lungs. If needed HRCT to be done separately.

2.6.3   PET Technique

After the CT is over PET is done. In whole body, the different bed positions vary from six to seven beds, but this varies depending on the height of the patient. Each bed position will have overlap due to the concept of misregistration between the CT and PET. Each bed position varies from 11 to 15 mm [25].

Once the PET is over then delayed images of CT abdomen are taking to evaluate the bowel loops, Urinary bladder, and pelvic pathologies.

2.7   Image Interpretation

PET images depict the amount of radiotracer uptake in particular tissue, which is basically the concentration of the radiotracer uptake. These are the uncorrected images which have to be converted to the corrected images. This has to be done by the CT data which is used to convert uncorrected images to corrected images. This attenuation correction is being done by the 511-keV photons that are passing

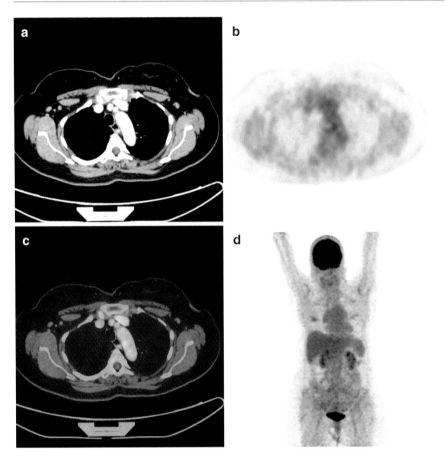

Fig. 2.1 Normal whole-body PET-CT scan from vertex of the skull to midthigh showing no abnormal physiological uptake. Normal physiological uptake seen in the renal pelvicalyceal system and urinary bladder

through the patient. Finally, corrected images of PET are ready. These fused images are reconstructed into Axial, Sagittal, and Coronal images (Figs. 2.1 and 2.2).

The different criteria for the assessment of the radiotracer uptake are done by visual inspection of SUV max and glucose metabolic rate. The most widely used are SUV max, which is semi-quantification for the amount of FDG uptake.

The normal physiological uptake is seen in the muscles and fat [26, 27]. Increased physiologic uptake is also seen in the brain and heart, especially more prominently seen in the cortex and basal ganglia in the brain. The uptake in the myocardium is based on the cardiac activity which appears normal and physiologic in the majority of whole-body scans. Dedicated cardiac scans are also done with FDG and other radiotracers. Mild uptake is also seen in the liver, spleen, and bone marrow, which can be physiological, systemic inflammation, and post-chemotherapy stages.

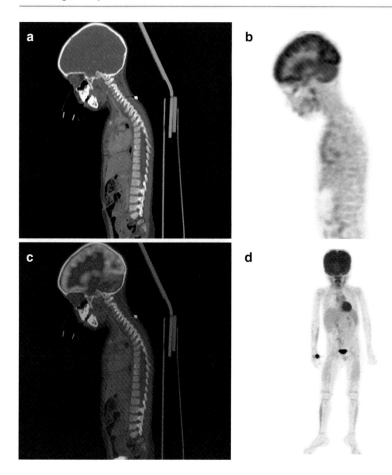

Fig. 2.2 Normal whole-body PET-CT scan from vertex of skull to feet. This is possible in the pediatric age group as examining PET-CT machine table is of sufficient height. Normal physiological uptake seen in the brain parenchyma, nasopharynx, cardia, and urinary bladder

Skeletal muscle uptake is also an important source of error, especially in cases where the patient is not resting or any involuntary activity is there (Fig. 2.3).

Physiological increase in FDG activity is also seen in the pelvicalyceal system of kidney and urinary bladder because FDG is excreted by the urinary system. Physiologic uptake also noted in the thyroid gland and GI tract. This physiologic uptake is highly variable which can be diffuse or focal can be seen in the all segments of the bowel, but most commonly seen in the caecum and recto-sigmoid junction. The role of CT with oral contrast in the bowel is more helpful, especially in relation to the mucosal or submucosal lesion, which can be malignant or premalignant. The SUV is a semiquantitative assessment of the radiotracer uptake from the static single point in the time PET image. The tissue tracer activity is in microcuries per gram, injected radiotracer dose in millicuries, and patient weight in

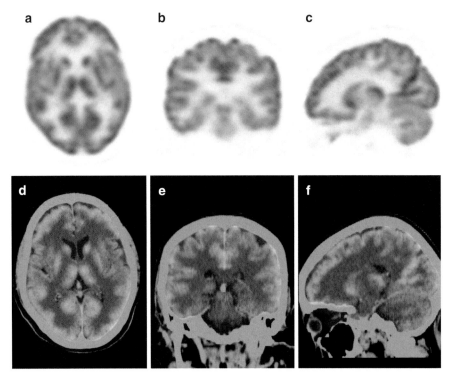

Fig. 2.3 Normal brain PET-CT uptake seen in the cerebral parenchyma. Cortex shows more uptake than the gray matter

kilograms. SUV of the tissue is documented as minimum, maximum, or mean in the region of interest (Figs. 2.4 and 2.5).

$$SUV = \frac{\text{Tracer activity in tissue}}{\text{Injected radiotracer dose / Patient weight}}$$

The tissue tracer activity is in microcuries per gram injected radiotracer dose is in millicuries per gram, injected radiotracer is in millicuries and patient weight is in kilograms.

The SUV values are quantified as minimum, maximum, and mean. The mean SUV is the mathematical mean of all the values. The minimum and maximum SUV max are the lowest and highest SUV max values. Ideally, the SUV max values are ranging from 0.5 to 2.5. Some of the literature mentions 2.5–3.0 and above SUV is consistent with the malignancy. But a lot of variations are there in this. It is better to have less radiotracer uptake. Variations are also seen in this which can be quantified or optimized [28].

With this, it is important to set a protocol for standardized SUV values.

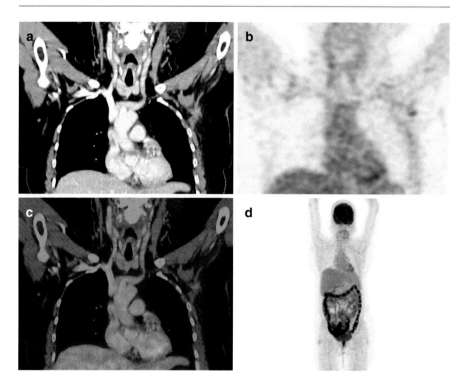

Fig. 2.4 Normal whole-body PET-CT scan with physiological uptake in the distal ileal loops and entire colon. This physiological uptake has to be differentiated from the pathological uptake in the bowel loops

Some of the studies we need to use special protocols like in the Head and Neck lesions Puff cheek technique is commonly used. This helps in the evaluation of the in situ lesions in buccal regions (Fig. 2.6). The other protocols like administration of the Lasix for the proper urinary bladder distension for small focal lesions or mild subtle urinary bladder wall thickening. Rectal contrast for the well distension of the anorectal, rectal, and sigmoid colon lesions. This is crucial for the well delineation of the focal, mild wall thickenings.

2.8   Limitations and Artifacts of PET-CT

Patient motion is the commonest cause of the artifacts. Proper PET and CT co-registration have to be done which is mostly based on the spatial resolution of the radiotracer activity and the attenuation correction. CT artifacts also caused by metallic artifacts and prosthesis, etc. will cause a lot of attenuation correction artifacts [29, 30]. Some other artifacts like significant activity before or after injecting the FDG.

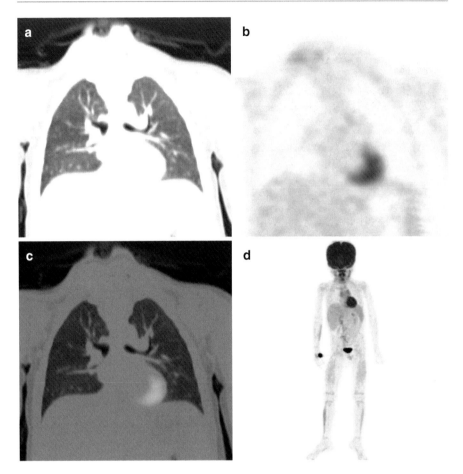

Fig. 2.5 Whole-body PET-CT scan of pediatric age group. Lung fields appear normal. Site of the injection of radiotracer seen at the right wrist joint. Normal physiological uptake seen in cerebral parenchyma, nasopharynx, cardia, and urinary bladder

Normal uptake should not be confused with physiologic uptake in kidney, brain, bowel, cardia, liver, and other organs.

2.9   Advantages of PET-CT

PET-CT is helpful in accurate localization of small radiotracer uptakes, distinguishing the normal and abnormal disease activities.

PET-CT combined imaging modality provides excellent functional information from PET and spatial and contrast resolution of the CT [31, 32].

PET-CT attenuation correction for quantitative or semiquantitative assessment of data which can be done by CT.

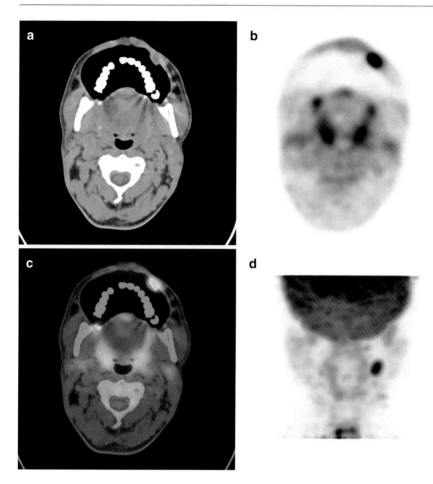

Fig. 2.6 Puff cheek technique is the specific technique that is helpful in differentiating the small subtle lesions and in situ lesions of buccal mucosa and also involving the gingivobuccal sulcus and retromolar trigone. Here in this small nodular lesion seen in the left buccal region is more clearly seen and shows significant uptake. This clarity of this lesion would be not precise if done in routine protocol

2.10 Conclusion

Thus, PET-CT is an important imaging modality, which has evolved in a significant way for imaging. The basis of the detection of the coincidence photons during annihilation, accurate co-registration of the quantitative and functional information with CT is the hallmark of the PET-CT imaging. Patient preparation, data acquisition, data reconstruction, and image interpretation are crucial to the high-quality PET-CT imaging. With many newer radiotracers and applications, it is the modality of choice in many conditions.

References

1. Mankoff DA. A definition of molecular imaging. J Nucl Med. 2007;48(6):18N, 21N.
2. Pichler BJ, Judenhofer MS, Pfannenberg C. Multimodal imaging approaches: PET/CT and PET/MRI—part 1. Handb Exp Pharmacol. 2008;185:109–32.
3. Mittra E, Quon A. Positron emission tomography/computed tomography: the current technology and applications. Radiol Clin N Am. 2009;47:147–60.
4. Ownsend DW, Carney J, Yap JT, Hall NC. PET/CT today and tomorrow. J Nucl Med. 2004;45(suppl):4S–14S.
5. van der Vos CS, Koopman D, Rijnsdorp S, Arends AJ, Boellaard R, van Dalen JA, et al. Quantification, improvement, and harmonization of small lesion detection with state-of-the-art PET. Eur J Nucl Med Mol Imaging. 2017;44(Suppl 1):4–16.
6. Slomka PJ, Pan T, Germano G. Recent advances and future progress in PET instrumentation. Semin Nucl Med. 2016;46:5–19.
7. Phelps ME, Hoffmann EJ, Mullani NA, et al. Application of annihilation coincidence detection to trans-axial reconstruction tomography. Nucl Med. 1975;16:210–24.
8. Omami G, Tamimi D, Barton F. Branstetter basic principles and applications of ^{18}F-FDG-PET/CT in oral and maxillofacial imaging: a pictorial essay. Imaging Sci Dent. 2014;44(4):325–32.
9. Synowiecki MA, Perk LR, Frank J, Nijsen W. Production of novel diagnostic radionuclides in small medical cyclotrons. EJNMMI Radiopharm Chem. 2018;3:3.
10. Peng H, Levin CS. Recent developments in PET instrumentation. Curr Pharm Biotechnol. 2010;11(6):555–71.
11. Vandenbroucke A, Foudray AMK, Olcott PD, Levin CS. Performance characterization of a new high-resolution PET scintillation detector. Phys Med Biol. 2010;55:5895–911.
12. Kułakowski A, et al. The contribution of Marie Skłodowska-Curie to the development of modern oncology. Anal Bioanal Chem. 2011;400(6):1583–6.
13. Shahhosseini S. PET radiopharmaceuticals. Iran J Pharm Res. 2011;10(1):1–2.
14. Tanaka S, Nishio T, Tsuneda M, et al. Improved proton CT imaging using a bismuth germanium oxide scintillator. Phys Med Biol. 2018;63(3):035030.
15. Berger A. Positron emission tomography. BMJ. 2003;326(7404):1449.
16. Lee JP, Ito M, Lee JS. Evaluation of a fast photomultiplier tube for time-of-flight PET. Biomed Eng Lett. 2011;1:174–9.
17. Dash A, Chakravarty R. Radionuclide generators: the prospect of availing PET radiotracers to meet current clinical needs and future research demands. Am J Nucl Med Mol Imaging. 2019;9(1):30–66.
18. Almuhaideb A, Papathanasiou N, Bomanji J. ^{18}F-FDG PET/CT imaging in oncology. Ann Saudi Med. 2011;31(1):3–13.
19. Shen B, Huang T, Sun Y. Revisit ^{18}F-fluorodeoxyglucose oncology positron emission tomography: "systems molecular imaging" of glucose metabolism. Oncotarget. 2017;8(26):43536–42.
20. Yamada T, Uchida M, Kwang-Lee K, et al. Correlation of metabolism/hypoxia markers and fluoro-deoxyglucose uptake in oral squamous cell carcinomas. Oral Surg Oral Med Oral Pathol Oral Radiol. 2012;113:464–71.
21. Kinahan PE, Fletcher JW. PET/CT standardized uptake values (SUVs) in clinical practice and assessing response to therapy. Semin Ultrasound CT MR. 2010;31(6):496–505.
22. Benamor M, Ollivier L, Brisse H, Moulin-Romsee G, et al. PET/CT imaging: what radiologists need to know. Cancer Imaging. 2007;7(Special issue A):S95–9.
23. Sprinz C, Zanon M, Altmayer S, et al. Effects of blood glucose level on 18F fluorodeoxyglucose (18F-FDG) uptake for PET/CT in normal organs: an analysis on 5623 patients. Sci Rep. 2018;8:2126.
24. Berthelsen AK, Holm S, Loft A, et al. PET/CT with intravenous contrast can be used for PET attenuation correction in cancer patients. Eur J Nucl Med Mol Imaging. 2005;32:1167–75.
25. Mawlawi O, Pan T, Macapinlac HA, et al. PET/CT imaging techniques, considerations, and artifacts. J Thorac Imaging. 2006;21(2):99–110.

26. Shammas A, Lim R, Charron M. Pediatric FDG PET/CT: physiologic uptake, normal variants, and benign conditions. Radiographics. 2009;29(5):1467–86.
27. Abouzied MM, Crawford ES, Nabi HA. 18F-FDG imaging: pitfalls and artifacts. J Nucl Med Technol. 2005;33(3):145–55.
28. Jennings M, Marcu LG, Bezak E. PET-specific parameters and radiotracers in theoretical tumour modeling. Comput Math Methods Med. 2015;2015:415923.
29. Freedenberg M, Badawi RD, Tarantal AF, et al. Performance and limitations of positron emission tomography (PET) scanners for imaging very low activity sources. Physica Med. 2014;30(1):104. https://doi.org/10.1016/j.ejmp.2013.04.001.
30. Pettinato C, Nanni C, Farsad M. Artifacts of PET/CT images. Biomed Imaging Interv J. 2006;2(4):e60.
31. Cazzato RL, Garnon J, Shaygi B, et al. PET/CT-guided interventions: indications, advantages, disadvantages and the state of the art. Minim Invasive Ther Allied Technol. 2018 Feb;27(1):27–32.
32. Ell PJ. The contribution of PET/CT to improved patient management. Br J Radiol. 2006;79:32–6.

Physiological Variants in PET-CT

3

Key Points

PET-CT is the hybrid imaging modality consisting of functional and anatomical imaging. In PET-CT, the common indication is in malignancy, but now a lot of the newer applications are being evaluated by this modality. A lot of physiological changes occur in our body and there are chances of false uptake due to these physiological changes.

3.1   Introduction

PET-CT is the functional imaging modality is commonly used for various indications. Now the role has extended for evaluation of various benign pathologies and one of the commonest is infection and inflammation. Abnormal uptake or increased uptake is one of the ways to differentiate and diagnose these pathologies. Many physiological uptakes are also seen and show significantly increased uptake which has a problem to differentiate with any associated pathologies. Various incidental findings are also seen in the various locations in the body that can be benign. This needs to be differentiated with the normal physiological and abnormal findings. Most important reasons are inflammation, infection, physiological variants, trauma, iatrogenic processes, and post-therapy changes [1, 2]. For this, the knowledge of the normal physiologic uptake is important and should be differentiated from the abnormal pathological uptakes.

F-18 FDG Fluorodeoxyglucose is commonly used radiotracer and the basis of the metabolism is the glucose metabolism. This is the basis of the FDG accumulation and metabolism in general [3, 4]. Glucose levels should be normal that is the important criterion.

3.2 Physiological Variants in FDG Radiotracer

3.2.1 Brain

Brain parenchyma glucose is an important metabolite for metabolism. Approximately 20% of total body glucose metabolism in the fasting state is seen in the brain parenchyma. The pattern of uptake in the normal brain and the aging brain has peculiar characteristics. This normal physiological uptake should not be considered as abnormal. Normally the physiological uptake will be bilateral and symmetrically common in basal ganglia, posterior cingulate cortex, and occipital cortex. Mildly reduced uptake seen in the medial temporal cortex. In resting state normal cerebral parenchyma, the gray to white matter activity ratio is 2.5–4.1. The cerebral metabolic rate values for glucose is approximately 15 μmol/min/100 g for white matter and 40–60 μmol/min/100 g for the gray matter (Fig. 3.1).

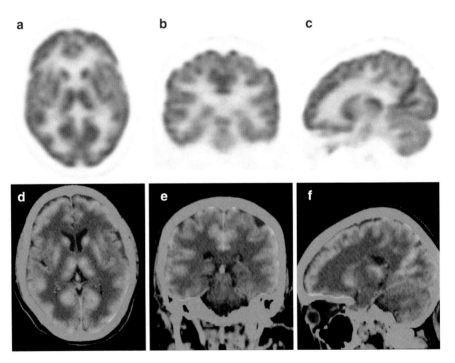

Fig. 3.1 Mild increase in uptake will be seen in the bilateral thalamus, globus pallidus, and putamen along with the cortical gray matter

3.2.2 Head and Neck

The normal lymphoid tissue is also another important area of normal physiological uptake of FDG. This physiologic uptake can be identified as the symmetric uptake on both sides. Major salivary glands and Laryngeal uptake, are having bilateral symmetrical uptake which is the important criteria to distinguish from pathological uptake. Patient movement shows increased muscle activity and can be seen in movement disorders, noncooperative patients, and other causes. Cervical spinal cord also shows minimal activity in the supine position. Very rarely thyroid also shows a mild increase uptake but the cause is not identified mostly physiological. Thus, FDG PET-CT plays an important role in the evaluation of various normal physiological uptake and variants [5] (Fig. 3.2).

3.2.3 Brown Fat

Brown adipose tissue acts as a thermogenic organ by producing heat to maintain the temperature of the body, especially in young. This is mostly related to non-shivering thermogenesis and diet-induced thermogenesis. With this capacity, this tissue has elevated cellular density, rich vascularization, innervations, and intracellular lipid components. This brown fat uses glucose as a source of adenosine triphosphate, which is required for fat metabolism and ultimately heat production. Thus, this fat will cause increased uptake due to the hypermetabolic activity. This is more commonly seen in the newborn and gradually diminishes as age increases. This is more common in women. The other areas where the brown fat uptake is in axillae, mediastinum, intercostals regions, paravertebral, and perinephric regions. PET-CT can easily identify physiological activity due to brown fat can be easily differentiated distinguished from pathological one [6] (Fig. 3.3).

3.3 Physiologic Uptake in Chest

3.3.1 Thymus

In pediatric age group, thymus is one of the common causes of physiological uptake. The reason is physical movements and emotional stress. This is not seen in adults. Thymic hyperplasia is one of the causes of increased uptake more likely reactive after post-therapy changes more commonly seen in the pediatric age group and young adults. Sometimes the thymic hyperplasia needs to be differentiated from physiological uptake. FDG PET-CT plays an important role in the evaluation of these various physiological uptakes in the thymus [7–9] (Fig. 3.4).

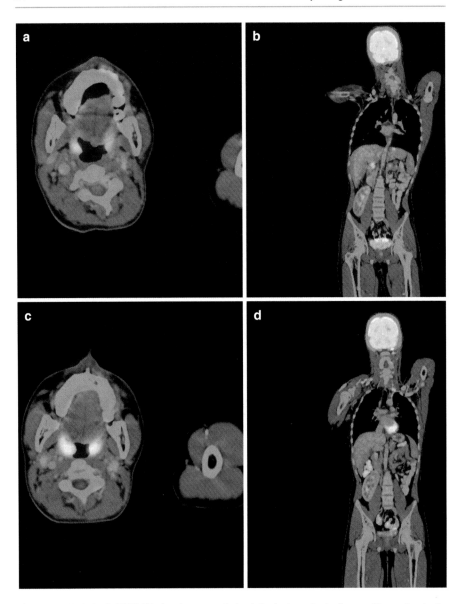

Fig. 3.2 Whole-body PET-CT showing normal physiological uptake in the tonsillar region in the neck and cardiac uptake

3.3.2 Myocardial Metabolism

Cardiac muscle's main metabolic agent is glucose. This activity is mostly seen in the left ventricle. Uptake in the other cardiac chambers is pathological. Cardiac muscle activity is also seen due to increase in metabolism. This must be differentiated from pathological uptake.

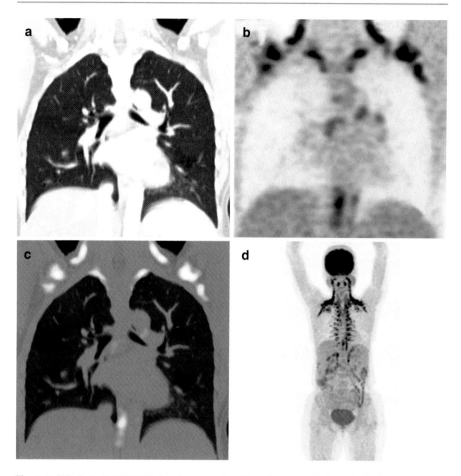

Fig. 3.3 Whole-body PET-CT showing irregular bilateral symmetrical uptake in the neck and in the chest wall due to brown fat

The myocardial metabolism depending on the fasting status can show the metabolism-related to fatty acids and glucose. FDG PET-CT plays an important role in the evaluation and differentiating the physiological and abnormal myocardial metabolisms [10, 11] (Fig. 3.5).

3.3.3   Breast Parenchyma

The hormonal changes can cause changes in the breast parenchyma. This is seen in the puberty and postmenopausal women. Increased uptake is also seen in the lactating breast parenchyma [12]. This uptake is mostly physiological uptake. The role of PET-CT is more defined to differentiate between the physiological and the pathological uptakes (Fig. 3.6).

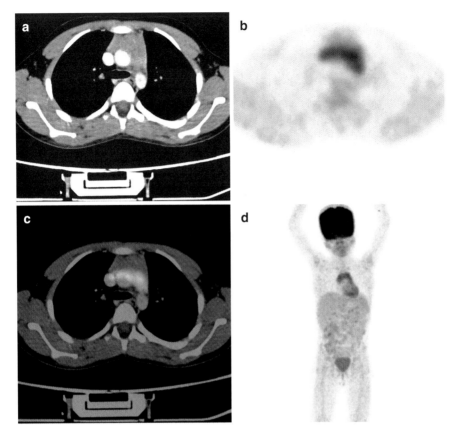

Fig. 3.4 Whole-body PET-CT showing the diffuse mild uptake in the thymus, otherwise also can be due to reactive changes due to post-chemotherapy changes

3.3.4   Lipomatous Hypertrophy

Increased amount of fat at the interatrial septum also shows increased uptake. Here FDG PET-CT plays an important role to differentiate between this physiological and pathological uptake [13].

3.4   Physiologic Uptake in the Abdomen

3.4.1   Bowel Loops

Physiological uptake is also seen in the bowel loops which needs most of the time CT correlation to confirm or rule out the pathology. If suspected, then delayed PET-CT to be taken to evaluate and quantify the pathologies [14]. The role of the CT here is to evaluate any minor changes such as mild wall thickening, adjacent fibrotic strands, or peritoneal thickening (Fig. 3.7).

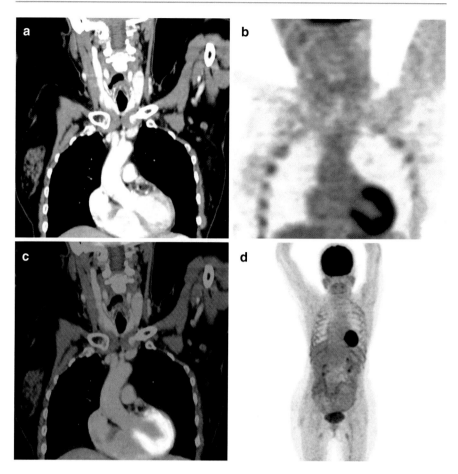

Fig. 3.5 (Normal cardiac uptake): Whole-body PET-CT showing normal physiological uptake in myocardium with no CT abnormality

3.4.2 Kidneys and Pelvicalyceal System

The physiological tracer uptake is seen in the kidneys and the pelvicalyceal system as radiotracer is being excreted through the kidneys. The various pathologies need to be differentiated from the physiological conditions by PET-CT [15, 16] (Fig. 3.8).

3.4.3 Urinary Bladder

The excretion of the radiotracer is through the kidneys and the tracer activity will be seen in the urinary bladder. If needed delayed scans to be taken and the Lasix can be given to evaluate the urinary bladder pathologies separately [17]. The role of Lasix is defined for the evaluation of focal wall thickening which will be differentiated from the partially distended urinary bladder.

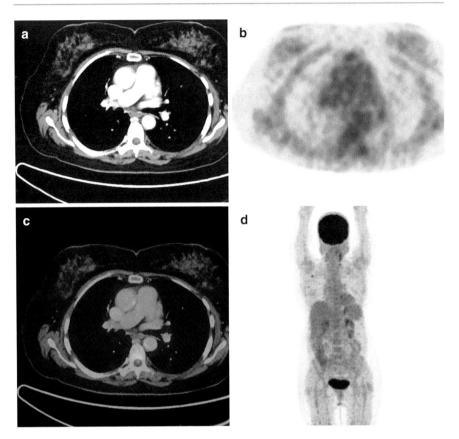

Fig. 3.6 Whole-body PET-CT at the level of bilateral breast showing minimal uptake in bilateral fibro-glandular tissue suggestive of normal physiological uptake in bilateral breast parenchyma

3.4.4   Ovarian Follice

Mild physiological uptake is seen in the ovarian follicle or corpus luteal cyst. This should not be confused with the abnormal uptake in other ovarian cysts with varied presentaions and labelled pathological [18] (Fig. 3.9).

3.5   Physiological Testicluar Uptake

Physiological uptake in the testes needs to be differentiated from pathological conditions, especially lymphoma and orchitis [19]. Again, the role of PET-CT is important.

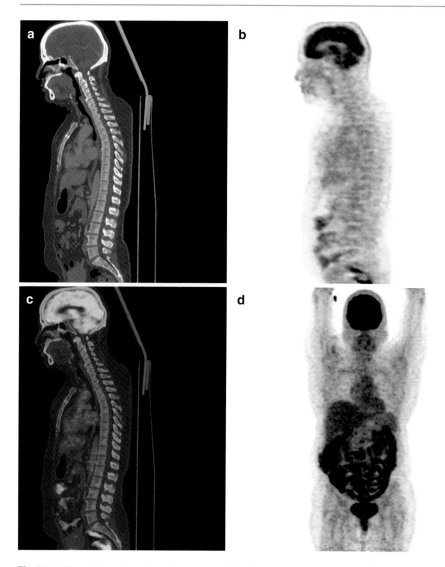

Fig. 3.7 (Normal bowel uptake): Whole-body PET-CT showing physiological FDG activity in the bowel loops with no corresponding CT abnormality

3.5.1 Bone Marrow

Reactive bone marrow also will show increased uptake. This is also seen in the post-therapy changes where diffuse increased uptake is seen without CT changes and needs to be differentiated from the marrow metastases (Fig. 3.10).

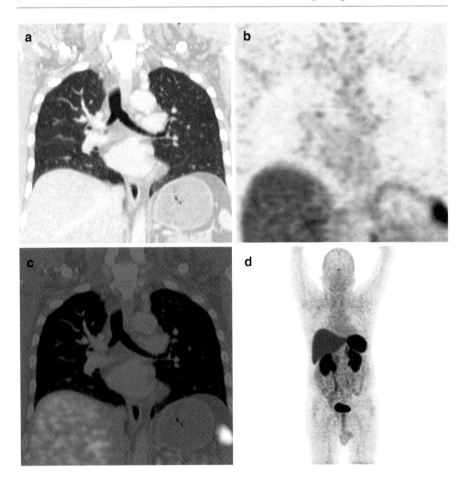

Fig. 3.8 Normal uptake of kidneys and pelvicalyceal system. Whole-body PET-CT DOTONAC scan showing intense FDG activity in both kidneys and pelvicalyceal system suggestive of normal physiological uptake. Also seen moderate metabolic activity in the liver. Spleen shows significant metabolic activity suggestive of physiological uptake

3.6   Physiological Uptake with DOTANOC and PSMA

Physiological diffuse increased uptake in the spleen, liver, and bowel [20]. Thus, some radiotracer affinity needs to be kept in mind before labelling it pathological (Fig. 3.11).

3.7   Physiological Uptake in Pediatric Patients

The normal distribution of the uptake in the pediatric age group is also seen in the same places except like thymus which is commonly seen [21].

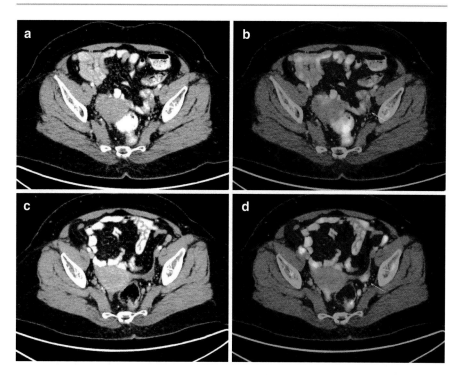

Fig. 3.9 Normal ovarian follicle uptake. PET-CT whole body at the level of pelvis showing tracer activity in the normal ovary with SUV max of 2.8 suggestive of physiological uptake

3.8   Technical Causes

The various technical causes that can be corrected are patient preparation, no physical movements or exercise, patient to be warm and relaxed, and no stress. Intravenous contrast administration will cause artifact related hot spots on PET [22, 23].

The other artifacts seen are metallic artifacts like dental clips, dental fillings metallic prosthesis, pacemaker, chemotherapy, and catheters (Figs. 3.12 and 3.13).

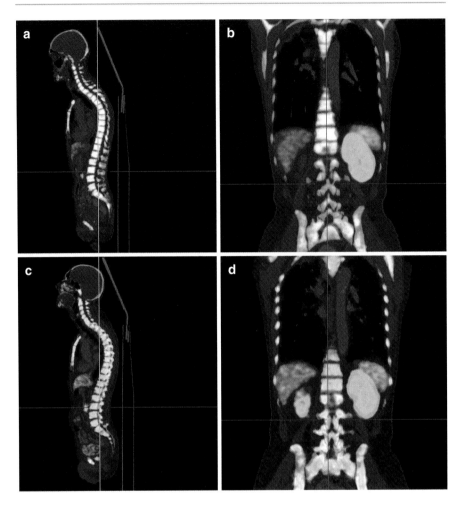

Fig. 3.10 Whole-body PET-CT showing diffuse increased uptake in the bone marrow of all the axial and appendicular skeleton due to physiological reactive changes and needs to be differentiated from the pathological marrow uptake. There is incidental mild uptake in the visualized right kidney and entire left kidney

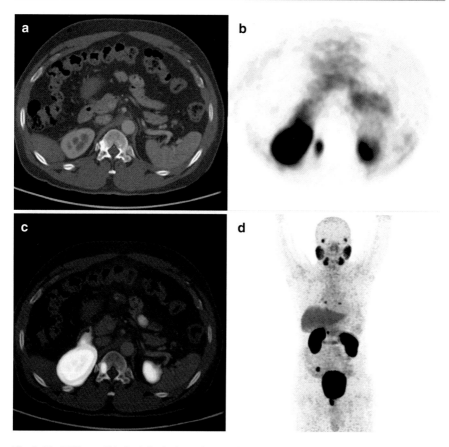

Fig. 3.11 Diffuse mild physiological uptake seen in the bilateral submandibular glands, bilateral sublingual glands, both kidneys, liver, and urinary bladder as described

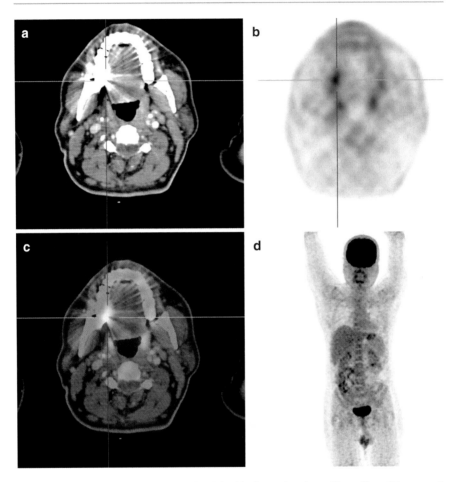

Fig. 3.12 Focal area of uptake seen on the right side due to dental metallic artifacts. These metallic artifacts uptake needs to be differentiated from the pathological uptake, especially from the associated infection of the artifact

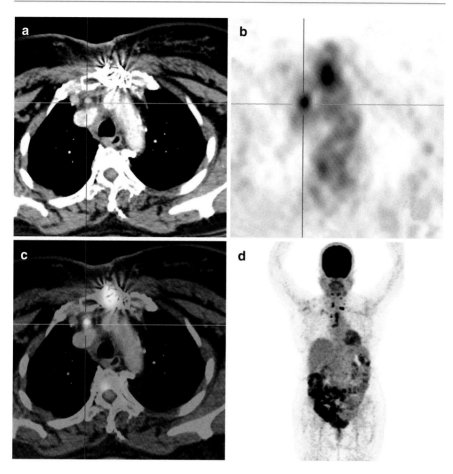

Fig. 3.13 Focal area of uptake seen in the sternum. These metallic artifacts uptake needs to be differentiated from the pathological uptake, especially from the associated infection of the artifact

3.9   Conclusion

Thus, physiological and pathological uptakes can be differentiated easily.

References

1. Cook GJ, Fogelman I, Maisey MN. Normal physiological and benign pathological variants of 18-fluoro-2-deoxyglucose positron-emission tomography scanning: potential for error in interpretation. Semin Nucl Med. 1996;26(4):308–14.
2. Cook GJ, Maisey MN, Fogelman I. Normal variants, artefacts and interpretative pitfalls in PET imaging with 18-fluoro-2-deoxyglucose and carbon-11 methionine. Eur J Nucl Med. 1999;26(10):1363–78.
3. Abouzied MM, Crawford ES, Nabi HA. 18F-FDG imaging: pitfalls and artifacts. J Nucl Med Technol. 2005;33(3):145–55; quiz 162–3.
4. Culverwell AD, Scarsbrook AF, Chowdhury FU. False-positive uptake on 2-[^{18}F]-fluoro-2-deoxy-D-glucose (FDG) positron-emission tomography/computed tomography (PET/CT) in oncological imaging. Clin Radiol. 2011;66(4):366–82. https://doi.org/10.1016/j.crad.2010.12.004.
5. Blodgett TM, Fukui MB, Snyderman CH, Branstetter BF, McCook BM, Townsend DW, Meltzer CC. Combined PET-CT in the head and neck: part 1. Physiologic, altered physiologic, and artifactual FDG uptake. Radiographics. 2005;25(4):897–912.
6. Truong MT, Erasmus JJ, Munden RF, Marom EM, Sabloff BS, Gladish GW, et al. Focal FDG uptake in mediastinal brown fat mimicking malignancy: a potential pitfall resolved on PET/CT. AJR Am J Roentgenol. 2004;183:1127–32.
7. Nguyen M, Varma V, Perez R, Schuster DM. CT with histopathologic correlation of FDG uptake in a patient with pulmonary granuloma and pleural plaque caused by remote talc pleurodesis. AJR Am J Roentgenol. 2004;182(1):92–4.
8. Murray JG, Erasmus JJ, Bahtiarian EA, Goodman PC. Talc pleurodesis simulating pleural metastases on 18F-fluorodeoxyglucose positron emission tomography. AJR Am J Roentgenol. 1997;168(2):359–60.
9. Brink I, Reinhardt MJ, Hoegerle S, Altehoefer C, Moser E, Nitzsche EU. Increased metabolic activity in the thymus gland studied with 18F-FDG PET: age dependency and frequency after chemotherapy. J Nucl Med. 2001;42(4):591–5.
10. Lobert P, Brown RK, Dvorak RA, Corbett JR, Kazerooni EA, Wong KK. Spectrum of physiological and pathological cardiac and pericardial uptake of FDG in oncology PET-CT. Clin Radiol. 2013;68:e59–71.
11. Ding HJ, Shiau YC, Wang JJ, Ho ST, Kao A. The influences of blood glucose and duration of fasting on myocardial glucose uptake of [18F]fluoro-2-deoxy-D-glucose. Nucl Med Commun. 2002;23:961–5.
12. Kumar R, Chauhan A, Zhuang H, et al. Standardized uptake values of normal breast tissue with 2-deoxy-2-[F-18]fluoro-D: −glucose positron emission tomography: variations with age, breast density, and menopausal status. Mol Imaging Biol. 2006;8:355–62.
13. Gerard PS, Finestone H, Lazzaro R, et al. Intermittent FDG uptake in lipomatous hypertrophy of the interatrial septum on serial PET/CT scans. Clin Nucl Med. 2008 Sep;33(9):602–5.
14. Ahmad Sarji S. Physiological uptake in FDG PET simulating disease. Biomed Imaging Interv J. 2006;2(4):e59.
15. Piccoli GB, Arena V, Consiglio V, et al. Positron emission tomography in the diagnostic pathway for intracystic infection in adpkd and "cystic" kidneys. A case series. BMC Nephrol. 2011;12:48.

16. Zincirkeser S, Sahin E, Halac M, et al. Standardized uptake values of normal organs on 18F-fluorodeoxyglucose positron emission tomography and computed tomography imaging. J Int Med Res. 2007;35:231–6.
17. Kitajima K, Nakamoto Y, Senda M, Onishi Y, Okizuka H, Sugimura K. Normal uptake of 18F-FDG in the testis: an assessment by PET/CT. Ann Nucl Med. 2007;21:405–10.
18. Demirci E, Sahin OE, Ocak M, et al. Normal distribution pattern and physiological variants of 68Ga-PSMA-11 PET/CT imaging. Nucl Med Commun. 2016;37(11):1169–79.
19. Shammas A, Lim R, Charron M. Pediatric FDG PET/CT: physiologic uptake, normal variants, and benign conditions. Radiographics. 2009;29(5):1467–86. https://doi.org/10.1148/rg.295085247.
20. Cook GJ, Wegner EA, Fogelman I. Pitfalls and artefacts in 18FDG PET and PET/CT oncologic imaging. Semin Nucl Med. 2004;34(2):122–33.
21. Todd M, Blodgett MD, Ajeet S, Mehta BS, Amar S, Mehta BS, et al. PET/CT artifacts. Clin Imaging. 2011;35(1):49–63.
22. Abouzied MM, Crawford ES, Nabi HA. 18 F-FDG imaging: pitfalls and artifacts. J Nucl Med Technol. 2005;33(3):145–55.
23. Hany TF, Heuberger J, Schulthess GK. Iatrogenic FDG foci in the lungs: a pitfall of PET image interpretation. Eur Radiol. 2003;13(9):2122–7.

Dual Time Point PET-CT Imaging

4

Key Points

(DTPI) Dual time point Imaging FDG PET-CT is the most widely used hybrid imaging modality for various applications with majority applications in oncology [1, 2]. The basis of the whole-body imaging is for identifying the infective focus, extent of disease, and monitoring response to therapy. There are various multiple causes of benign uptake on PET. The degree of FDG uptake is directly proportional to metabolic rate and number of glucose transporters. The concept of FDG uptake in tumors is based on the increase in the number of glucose transporters in malignant cells. However, many pathologies including infection inflammation also show increased glucose transporters. This has to be differentiated from malignant pathologies [3–5]. This has become the basis of increased FDG uptake in any metabolically active lesions, which can be malignant or nonmalignant entities.

4.1 Introduction

What is dual point imaging? The dual point imaging is delayed imaging after the first routine PET-CT imaging protocol and used to differentiate the inflammatory and malignant processes. This is used to enhance the sensitivity of the PET-CT scan. The concept of this that the FDG uptake at the second or third acquisitions the variabilities in the uptake can differentiate between the malignant and nonmalignant lesions. This delayed imaging can be from 90 to 270 min from the primary PET imaging [6–8]. The basic concept here is SUV value increases over time in malignant lesions due to the capability of malignant cells to retain the tracer contrast due to increased glucose metabolism. Where is SUV values are stable or decreases in benign pathology because the glucose metabolism is reduced as the time is increased. With this concept, FDG PET as significantly improved specificity and sensitivity.

© The Author(s), under exclusive license to Springer Nature
Singapore Pte Ltd. 2021
S. Shaikh, *PET-CT in Infection and Inflammation*,
https://doi.org/10.1007/978-981-15-9801-2_4

The usefulness of PET-CT is based on staging, monitoring response to therapy, and relapse of the disease. The most widely used radiotracer is fluorodeoxyglucose (FDG). The basis of uptake in inflammatory conditions is the affinity of glucose transporters for deoxyglucose which will be apparently increased by various cytokines and growth factors. The concept of FDG uptake in infections is related to granulocytes and mononuclear cells using a large quantity of glucose by hexose monophosphate shunt.

With the increasing use of FDG PET, there is also increasing mention of nonspecific FDG uptake in multiple sides of varying a wide spectrum of anatomical and physiological processes. With this, the benign lesions also show increased FDG uptake with false-positive results and decreased positive predictive value of PET and PET-CT in such settings. The SUV max of 2.5 is usually the reference for differentiating malignant from benign lesions [3, 9, 10]. However, there is a significant overlap of findings between the uptakes of malignant and benign lesions. The basic concept of increased FDG in malignant lesions for several hours after the injection of radiotracer is the affinity of the malignant cells to continuously trap FDG and retain contrast. This has to be differentiated from benign lesions. In one of the studies which showed FDG tracer distribution of radiotracer uptake in inflammatory lesions gradually increases up to 60 min postinjection of radiotracers and then decreases significantly. This hypothesis is important to differentiate between malignant and benign, malignant and inflammatory, and concurrent malignant and inflammatory lesions with relation to FDG tracer uptake [11, 12]. These malignant lesions show increased tracer uptake with time while in the non malignant lesions there is decrease in radiotracer. One of the studies with 29 patients with soft tissue masses were evaluated using a 6-h protocol consisting of 2-h dynamic acquisitions immediately after tracer injection. The histological evaluation of these lesions showed 17 benign lesions and 12 soft tissue lesions. This was the data of Hamberg et al. [13]. This showed that in some cases of malignant lesions take longer time after FDG injection to see the maximum standardized uptake.

4.2   Dual Time Point Imaging Protocol

Normal dynamic changes of uptake depend on various factors like tracer distribution time and plasma levels. As time precedes the background activity decreases with time and thus contrast between the target and the surrounding tissues becomes more obvious. Thus, the SUV values depend on the time elapsed between the administration of FDG and the image acquisition. With this, there is no exact timeline for the interpretation of the PET images to differentiate. But this knowledge is necessary to understand the dynamics of FDG uptake and analyze at different time limits in dual point delayed imaging.

There are different protocols that showed the various image acquisitions between 0 and 40 min, 1.5 h and 3 h after radiotracer injection. But no clear-cut demarcation is there for this evaluation. Another concept of tumor to non-tumor evaluation and tumor-to-organ ratio evaluation resulted in significantly higher amount of uptakes for 3 h compared with 1.5-h images. Thus, the tumor contrast and radiotracer uptake show different variabilities depending on the different protocols. One of the studies by Hustinx et al. [14] showed the significance of dual point imaging to differentiate between malignancy, inflammation, and normal tissues in the head and neck cancers. They studied 21 patients whoever submitted to PET and 70 min and then at 98 min, with a mean interval between scans of 28 min. Region of interest (ROI) was drawn on FDG focus which showed significantly increased uptake compared with a contralateral location at same level, especially in cases of tongue, larynx, and cerebellum to measure initial SUVs and changes over time for both pathological and normal structures. These preliminary results showed that the pattern of tumor uptake cannot be differentiated from normal and inflamed tissues, especially in this setting of the head and neck pathologies.

One of the important aspects to differentiate between temporal changes in FDG uptake and postoperative changes after surgery is difficult to be evaluated. However, with this dual point imaging technique, a significant amount of differentiation can be done by this technique. One of the studies with solitary pulmonary nodules on CT was conducted [15–17]. This study shows different SUV max starting from 60 min post-injection to multiple delayed imaging like SUV1, SUV2, SUV3, and SUV4 and further delayed imaging. Here the relevance of increased SUV between the first and the second PET scans, the quantification of no change or increase to be noted. SUV2 and SUV3 again no change or increase or decrease to be documented then further SUV3 and SUV4 delayed scans also needs to be evaluated. They studied 255 patients' primary PET after 60 min of FDG PET injection, second FDG PET 100 min after the injection. Second delay varying from any specified time for a particular pathology. Here, of 255 patients 265 SPNs were evaluated and 72 (27%) proved to be malignant and 193 patients (73%) benign. In this assessment of FDG PET-CT sensitivity, specificity, and accuracy were following for first primary PET scan 97, 58, and 68%. Then first delay 65, 92, and 85%, second delay 90, 80, and 83%, third delay 84, 91, and 89%, and fourth delay 84, 95, and 92%. Thus, the results obtained are based on these different criteria which show the benefit of dual point imaging in improving the sensitivity, specificity, and accuracy of these lesions. One of the biggest fallacies for evaluating these lung nodules shows no significant change or minimal changes in SUV values of inflammation, tuberculosis, sarcoidosis, and fungal infections. However, there is some relevance of information that is diagnosed by these particular newer protocols [18, 19] (Figs. 4.1 and 4.2).

4.3 Application of Dual Point Imaging

The dual point FDG PET-CT is recommended for staging lung cancer and differentiating between metastatic and nonmetastatic lesions [20, 21]. This technique has same relevance in the evaluation of regional lymph nodes in doubtful cases of known primary malignancy or concurrent malignant and nonmalignant lesions. The latter one is more difficult to differentiate but with the hypothetical analysis of delayed imaging it can be differentiated. The FDG uptake has to be reduced in cases

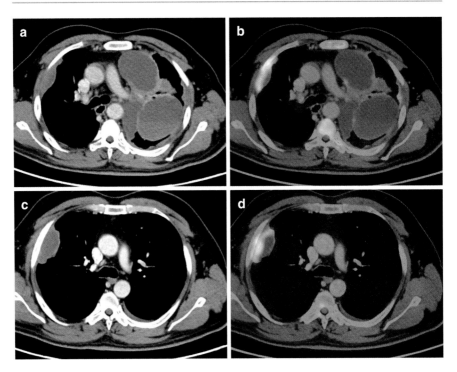

Fig. 4.1 Routine PET-CT scan showing focal right costal nodular pleural thickening with associated small loculated effusion. The SUV max was 9.6

of benign lesions in comparison with malignant lesion. Second, the difference in again SUV max between the different delayed images like first delayed, second delayed, and third delayed scans, this difference is important for quantification of various lesions. This hypothesis is of relevance in all the malignant lesions of all the organs except with some lesions that are not nearly differentiated, especially in low-grade neoplastic lesions (Figs. 4.3 and 4.4).

The SUV max mentioned usually reaches maximum levels after several hours but in some cases, it does not reach. The ideal time of the SUV to reach maximum levels starts from 45 to 60 min and has been reported to pause significantly under estimation of the true SUV value.

4.4   Dual Point Time Imaging in Musculoskeletal Imaging

4.4.1   Applications

The dual point technique mentioned above has relevance with the same protocol used for any lesions. The little drawback for these musculoskeletal lesions is the limitation to distinguish between or having a significant overlap between postoperative changes, residual disease, post-chemotherapy changes, post-radiation changes,

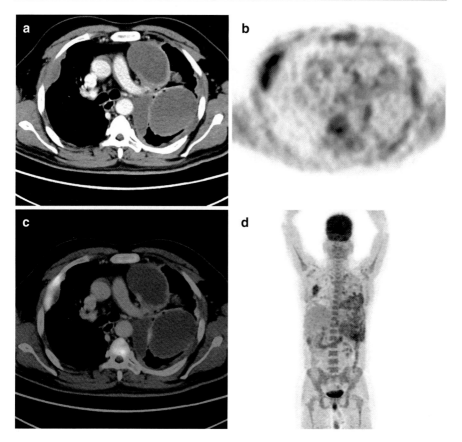

Fig. 4.2 The same case after 1 h delayed scan the SUV max value is 8.3. This shows that this focal nodular pleural thickening is more likely infective due to fall in the SUV values

and posttreatment changes in cases of nonmalignant pathologies. The muscular uptake also depends on adjacent edema, altered soft tissue planes and fibrosis. One of the important differentiating factors here is the muscle involvement with benign lesions and infective inflammatory lesions. Sometimes, it is difficult to differentiate between the various early grade of tumor vs. low-grade neoplastic muscular involvement [22]. One of the important aspects here is the SUV max cut off which is usually 2.4 differentiates between benign and malignant lesions [22–24]. One of the studies showed a different meta-analysis in the diagnosis of soft tissue lesions of muscle and found overall sensitivity, specificity, accuracy, positive predictive value, and negative predictive value for various differential diagnosis of soft tissue lesions to be 96%, 77%, 88%, 86%, and 90%, respectively. Other false-positive results in muscular benign lesions are diffuse tenosynovial joint cell tumor, hibernoma, sarcoidosis, myositis ossificans, abscesses, and inflammation. The false-negative results are due to myxoid liposarcomas, low-grade fibromyxoid sarcoma, well-differentiated liposarcomas, and spindle cell tumors [25]. Shin et al. [26] found a

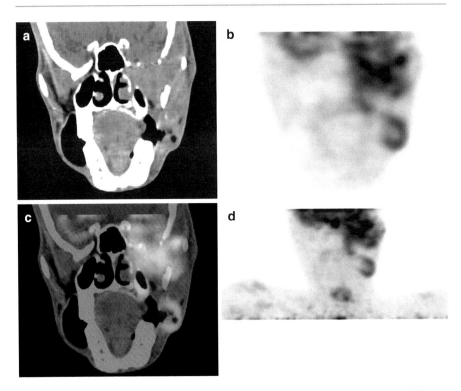

Fig. 4.3 The ill-defined lesion in the left maxillary region in the coronal CT image (**a**), PET image (**b**) and (**d**), and fused PET-CT (**c**) images showing the infiltrative lesion with SUV max of 7.8. This was the postoperative case of left buccal region carcinoma. Came for follow up for residual lesion

statistically significant difference in SUV max between the benign (Mean SUV max of 4.7) for benign soft tissue lesion and mean SUV max of 5.1 for benign bony lesions and malignant mean SUV max of 8.8. The sensitivity, specificity, and diagnostic accuracy were 80%, 65.2%, and 73%, respectively, with the total cut off of SUV max of 3.8. Some benign lesions like giant cell tumors, Langerhans cell histiocytosis, osteoblastoma are categorized as histiocytic or giant cell containing lesions. The higher uptake of FDG in nonmalignant lesions like fibrous dysplasia, fibroblasts, and other lesions characterized by cellular infiltrates, granuloma formation, and macrophage proliferations resulting in increased glycolysis. Some lesions like eosinophilic granuloma and tuberculosis, which have remarkably high FDG uptake also cannot be differentiated as per the study conducted by Aoki et al. These lesions cannot be distinguished from malignant lesions.

1. In one of the studies published in literature showed the role of 18F FDG PET or PET-CT in musculoskeletal tumors may found that the number of cases in each report which was insufficient to distinguish the exact patterns and characteristics of FDG uptake especially in benign lesions. This is one of the reason for low incidence in musculoskeletal lesions and limitation in using PET-CT for various

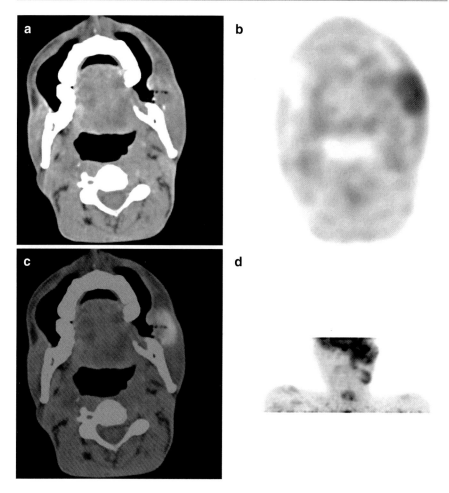

Fig. 4.4 This lesion is described in the Fig. 4.3 after 1 h delayed PET-CT scan showing metabolic activity with SUV max of 7.3. This minimal fall in the SUV max values is of not much relevance but histopathologically it turned out to be infective lesion secondary to postoperative changes. Thus, it is very difficult to differentiate between the benign and the malignant lesions, especially in minimal changes in the SUV max values. Here histopathological finding is of much relevance

    soft tissue and bone lesions because of cost-effectiveness issues and ethical considerations [27].

2. In FDG PET-CT studies, the differential diagnosis is not much of relevance as compared to conventional imaging because the conventional imaging uses more information about the structural changes.

3. The problem with PET-CT is nonuniform equipment various examination protocols varying postinjection scan times, anatomical methods, patient habitus, and other variations in SUV max for evaluation. These are difficulties where SUV max values will vary and this is more of relevance in the borderline cases of SUV max uptake where the consistent diagnosis has to be made but due to this lot of variations will be there.

4. The varied presentations of musculoskeletal lesions from aggressive to nonaggressive lesions, benign to malignant lesions, low- to high-grade lesions, and various histopathological subtypes, size of the lesions, tumor differentiation, and other parameters. Even though, the dual point imaging has a lot of variations and various musculoskeletal pathology.

4.4.2 Dual Point Imaging in Musculoskeletal Lesions: Clinical Results

In one of the prospective studies conducted by Tian et al. [28], 67 patients who had detected bone lesions by CT and MRI were included with an aim of differentiating benign vs. malignant and to determine the efficacy of FDG PET-CT. SUV values were measured from early and delayed images (SUV maxe and SUV maxd, respectively). Retention index was calculated who know the amount of tracer retention by the following formula. RI (percentage = $100\% \times$ (SUV maxd) − SUV maxe/SUV maxe. Both these parameters were compared between benign and malignant lesions. The differences in the SUV maxe were calculated and at some point considerable overlap was also seen between benign and malignant lesions. The sensitivity, specificity, and accuracy were 96%, 44%, and 72.4%, respectively. The PPV and NPV were 67.1% and 90.9%, respectively. In the second part of analysis in the study, there was a difference in the RI between benign and malignant lesions. By this method, the mean retention index was lower 7 ± 11 for benign lesions and $18 \pm$ for malignant lesions. Thus, RI cut off was tentatively achieved showing RI < 10 more likely benign, RI > 10 more likely to malignant. With this study, the sensitivity, specificity, and accuracy were 90.6%, 76%, and 83.7%, respectively. The PPV and NPV were 81.4% and 87.1%, respectively. Thus, this protocol is recommended for use of (DTPI) 18F FDG PET technique in the evaluation of various bone lesions.

One of the studies showed the amount of radiotracer uptake with malignant bony lesions and chronic osteomyelitis [27]. The SUV max and mean after 30- and 90-min postinjections were also evaluated by SUV max and SUV mean values. The median SUV and mean SUV have to be evaluated at some point. At some point, SUV max and SUV mean were evaluated in all malignant patients. And these values were significantly increased in the malignant lesions. However, the differentiation between the effective lesions like osteomyelitis and bone lesions cannot be differentiated in most of the cases. The phase of osteomyelitis also shows a varied amount of uptake, especially more in acute osteomyelitis and less in chronic osteomyelitis. By this dual point imaging, the various causes of spondylodiscitis can also be evaluated.

4.4.3 PET-CT Imaging Criteria for the Chest and Musculoskeletal Lesions

In most of the DTPI studies, early and delayed acquisitions were performed at I or II delayed scans. There was a significant variation in the DTPI during the evaluation in the delayed phase. Some variations were short between initial and delayed scans of 30 min various others there having quite long intervals of 120–140 min. This variation could be one of the major problems for the varying results. As mentioned above, the RI value varies significantly from the various criteria indicating the malignancy or infection inflammation. Lot of Potential for DTPI 18F FDG PET scan for differentiating and charecterising lesions. With the above-described protocols, the various results of PET imaging for differentiating between malignant and infective inflammatory lesions can be done to majority of extent. This dual point imaging has the potential role to provide this important and precise information. The background radiotracer uptake is also an important advantage of DTPI that can lead to various improved image contrast for detecting various pathologies. One of the fallacies, as described, is again based on the aggressiveness of benign tumors which may demonstrate an increase in 18F FDG uptake. This active infective inflammatory pathology is a major challenge to be distinguished in oncological setting. With so much of advancements still 18F FDG uptake in active inflammation and granulomatous lesions remains a limitation for accurate interpretation and differentiating from the other pathologies especially with the prevalence of coexisting malignancy and active infection. The differentiation between these two cannot be defined clearly. Now another debate is to differentiate active (acute) inflammation vs. inactive (chronic) inflammation. Another thing is of active granulomatous lesions vs. inactive granulomatous lesions vs. benign lesions (Figs. 4.5 and 4.6).

The lesion heterogenicity is also important for different histological subtypes and variants like different stromal matrix, vascularity, size of the lesion, genotyping, and immune status. With this, a lot of limitations are there which characterize the amount of radiotracer activity and the impact after therapy. There will also be a small issue related to normal tissues, which can have a different background activity. Sometimes difficult to evaluate, especially when the size of the lesion is small and not defined clearly. Any doubt at this point of evaluation should be rescanned and reevaluated to confirm or rule out a particular pathology. Small issue is also seen in obese patients or patients with systemic diseases like renal failure and diabetes. In these types of patients, delayed scan is of more relevance to occult lesions (Figs. 4.7 and 4.8).

With the limitation of conventional imaging techniques and F FDG radiotracer avidity many newer radiotracers or under trial 125 or I FIAU radiolabeled are used and supposed to be having affinity toward bacterial infections. This radiotracers helps in determining the challenges of infections that are difficult to diagnose because of nonspecific symptoms such as pain, arthritis, trauma, recent surgery, or in cases of aseptic loosening of prosthetic joint. Even various other radionuclide scans also cannot diagnose these conditions. The basis of FIAU PET-CT is based on amino acid metabolism. The scanning protocol of this FIAU PET-CT is post injection 2 and 24 h. This radiotracer is used for various clinical applications like known diabetes, knee joint replacement, to evaluate prosthesis infection, changes in laboratory parameters like CRP values, post-traumatic pain or non-united fractures, longstanding osteomyelitis, nonhealing venous ulcers, any joint swellings with pain, and associated degenerative changes in the joints along with the normal radiotracer

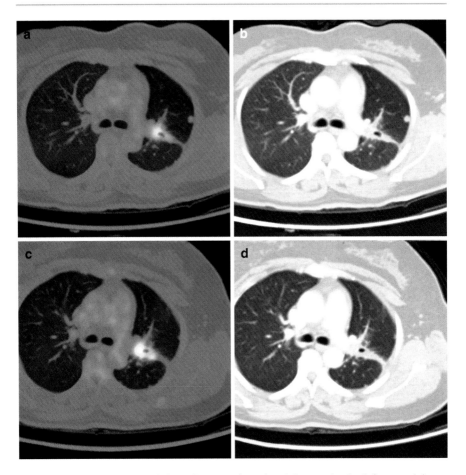

Fig. 4.5 Hypermetabolic small irregular parenchymal nodule seen in the left upper lobe on PET-CT with SUV max of 8.6

bio-distribution. The normal bio-distribution of this radiotracer has to be evaluated and known because this radiotracer is excreted by renal excretion. This FIAU radiotracer has little side effects of toxicity. Hepatotoxicity is one of the commonest ones. These PET findings also need to be verified by positive cultures, blood cells, or any associated infections. The infection can be focused on any region but the concurrent minimal uptake in the lungs and brain needs to be known before labeling its pathological uptake. This new radiotracer is now widely used for the evaluation of infection and inflammatory lesions along with other clinical findings and routine laboratory investigations.

With this advent, many infections with their focussed anatomical locations and sites can be easily evaluated and radiolabeled. Thus, this technique has become a unique approach in the evaluation of the infections which has limitations by FDG PET and other anatomical modalities (Figs. 4.9 and 4.10).

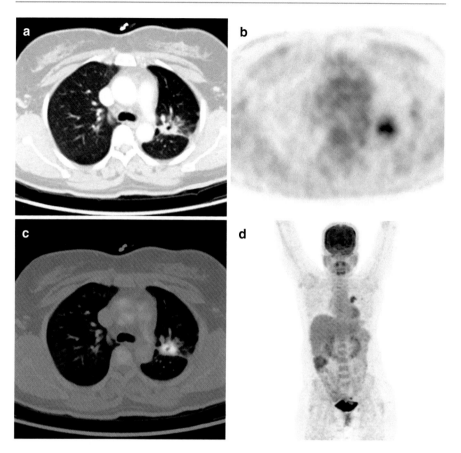

Fig. 4.6 This lesion on delayed scan showing a mild decrease in the metabolic activity with SUV max of 8.0 goes in favor of infective pathology

4.5   Dual Point Imaging in Abdominal Pathology

The concept of dual point imaging also applies to all the organs and systems in the abdomen.

4.5.1   Dual Point Imaging in Gastrointestinal Pathologies

GI infective inflammatory pathologies are one of the important pathological entities as their incidence and mortality in the last couple of years are significantly reduced. The early detection by 18F FDG as definitive improvement for these focal or local inflammatory changes is important. Many conventional imaging modalities has limited sensitivity and accuracy. Again, these findings are based

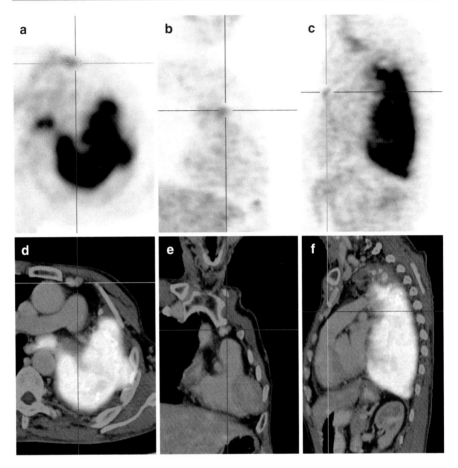

Fig. 4.7 Large hypermetabolic lesion in the entire left lung parenchyma with an SUV max of 13.6

on lesion size, lesion characterization, location, and histopathological status. With this, some studies tried to explore gastric distensions by giving nonionic oral contrast. PET-CT does not have much overall advantage compared to routine conventional studies, for example, in a focal gastric wall thickening which has to be evaluated, the first of foremost criteria is to distend the GI tract with oral contrast so that any subtle focal lesions can be better evaluated. Here FDG PET-CT has a role confined to the metabolic activity, amount of uptake, extent of the uptake, and any loco-regional involvement. The ideal method for this GI evaluation is fasting for at least 6 h and blood sugar levels should be <150. As already mentioned, FDG PET has less sensitivity compared to other imaging modalities like endoscopy, endoscopic ultrasound, and CT. PET-CT also has limitations in resolution, sensitivity, and accuracy. Usually, the commonest gastric pathology in the stomach is gastritis, gastric ulcers, and other rare infective inflammatory pathologies. The only biggest advantage here will be to differentiate between the

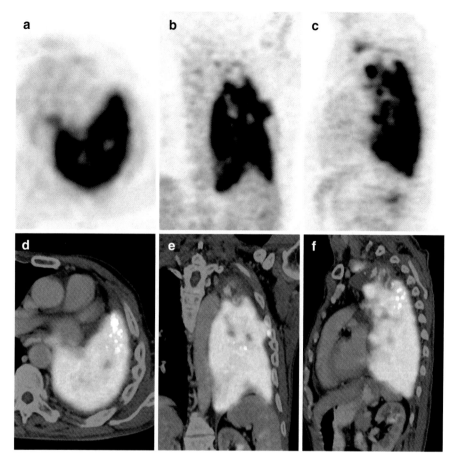

Fig. 4.8 Same lesion showing slight increase in the SUV max of 14.5. This doesn not go in favor of infective inflammatory pathology

benign and the malignant gastric ulcers depending on the amount of the uptake. Here again with delayed point imaging, the differentiation can be done easily. The various considerations of relatively large sensitivity with PET-CT depend on the newer techniques like 3D PET with CT gastrography. In one of the studies, the sensitivity on early imaging was 65.2% and AUC was only 0.635, i.e., 95%, CI. 0.507–0.764. With these results, it is little difficult to distinguish benign from malignant pathologies. The important concept of DTPI is the amount of uptake and the amount of clearance between IV FDG administration and imaging. One of the important advantages also is reduced normal background activity, which may increase FDG uptake in delayed imaging.

Thus, DTPI PET-CT plays an important significant role in differentiating benign from malignant lesions, benign vs. infective inflammatory lesions, and characterization of infective and inflammatory lesions.

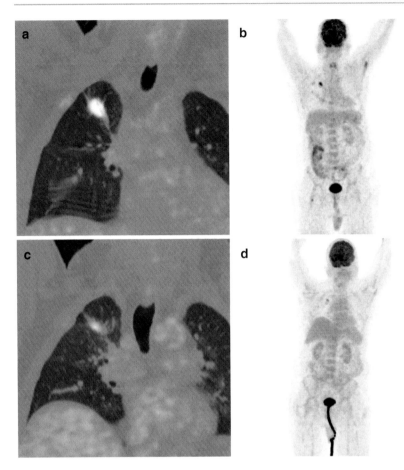

Fig. 4.9 Whole-body PET-CT with sections at the level of chest showing nodular lesion in right upper lobe with significant metabolic activity of 6.7 and in first delayed scan after 60 min it showing similar SUV max of 6.6. This feature does not represent any conclusive evidence. Biopsy reveals tuberculosis

4.5.2   Hepatobiliary Pathologies

The various infective inflammatory lesions that compete with malignant etiology are chronic organized liver abscess vs. cystic metastatic lesions [29, 30]. Infiltrative cholangitis is a discrete lesion or multifocal small lesions that can mimic cholangio-carcinoma. Diffuse metabolic infiltration of liver vs. diffuse malignant infiltration in cases of hematological malignancies.

Focal gall bladder wall thickening/diffuse cholecystitis has to be differentiated from focal gall bladder carcinoma or diffuse infiltrative gall bladder carcinoma [31]. Again, the pericholecystic infiltration needs to be differentiated cholangiocarci-noma vs. impacted sludge with cholangitis. All inflammatory lesions are associated

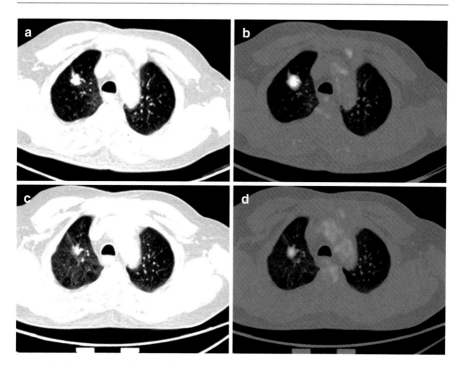

Fig. 4.10 Whole-body PET-CT with sections at the level of chest showing nodular lesion in right upper lobe with significant metabolic activity of 6.7 and in first delayed scan after 60 min it showing similar SUV max of 6.6. This feature does not represent any conclusive evidence. Biopsy reveals tuberculosis

with autoimmune status involving hepatobiliary regions. All the above-mentioned possible lesions have to be differentiated from each other as the entire management and planning and response to therapy are different. Here, dual point imaging plays a significant role in differentiating the above pathologies.

4.5.3   Pancreas

This is one of the commonest abdominal pathologies where FDG PET or proton of PET is useful in differentiating the focal area of pancreatitis with the focal small primary neoplastic lesion. With conventional imaging modalities, we cannot differentiate between these two pathologies but FDG PET-CT/proton of PET-CT can easily differentiate and distinguish any pancreatic malignancy which superadded pancreatitis. Pseudocyst of pancreas vs. cystic neoplastic lesions like serous and mucinous lesions involving the primary pancreas [32–34]. With this pathology, first of all, PET-CT can be used meticulously and in any doubtful cases. Delayed PET-CT imaging plays an important role and can be used frequently.

4.5.4 Spleen

Diffuse increased FDG uptake in the spleen is also the important hallmark of infective inflammatory diseases, especially tropical diseases like malaria. The diffuse increase uptake is also seen in the lymphoma or fungal infections or diffuse splenic metastases or sometimes reactive changes, but the relevance is in relation to infective inflammatory pathologies. Autoimmune diseases also show multiple organ involvement and helpful for diagnosis correlating the findings. The spleen as an organ has important functions of filtering the blood, monitoring the blood-borne antigens, leukocytes in the spleen include various subjects of TNB cells, dendritic cells, and macro phases. Recent analysis shows the metabolism of spleen is different in different pathologies, for example, autoimmune and localized infections. The hypothesis is different. Here FDG PET helps in differentiating the autoimmune and localized infections [35]. Splenic SUV value is obtained separately compared to bone marrow. The spleen-to-liver ratio of SUV is also a relevant finding for evaluating the tracer uptake. The other commonly involved pathologies in spleen are hemophagocytic lymphohistiocytosis, systemic lupus erythromatosis, chikikuchi disease, adult-onset still disease, vasculitis, or rheumatoid arthritis. As spleen is the largest lymphatic organ,. The spleen has no afferent lymph vessels, but only efferent lymph vessels. Here the spleen function is to monitor blood for microorganism and blood cells. As compared to lymph nodes who monitor lymphatic for local inflammation. The evaluation of spleen by F-FDG is to demonstrate the exact immunometabolism in systemic inflammations. Sepsis is the clinical entity with diffuse uptake in spleen and bone marrow with febrile patients. The diagnosis of sepsis is based on clinical presentation, vital signs, and identification of microorganisms, which are beyond in research. The diffuse uptake in the spleen is due to diffuse infiltrative patterns in the splenic parenchyma, the best example is lymphoma from increased splenic uptake. Bone marrow is also involved in systemic inflammation along with the spleen. The role of bone marrow is hematopoietic progenitor cell productions, where is spleen is the site of interaction of activated immune cells. The uptake in spleen also depends on the ferritin levels and splenic glucose metabolism.

4.5.5 Renal

The dual point imaging in renal pathologies is also significant relevance. These renal pathologies are described in a separate chapter.

With the newer imaging modality PET-MR lot of changes in evaluation will be there especially in relation to the soft tissue and muscle characterizations. However, the PET evaluation will be the same as that of PET-CT. However, the advancements in PET technicalities and radiotracer developments will have more impact in the future.

4.5.6 Inflammatory Bowel Diseases

Inflammatory bowel diseases comprise two important entities Crohn's disease and ulcerative colitis. Clinically they resemble each other. Both are chronic with relaxing inflammation, but they differ in the extent and pattern of involvement. Conventional imaging is commonly used but the accuracy is not sensitive, especially in relation to the inflammation. FDG PET-CT plays an important role in the evaluation of the early inflammatory changes that are not detected by any other modalities [36, 37]. The IBD also a diagnostic challenge, especially in children and adults in the early stages with episodes of flare-up. One of the studies shows the relevance of pediatric IBD, PET imaging is having better results compared to other conventional modalities. As shown in the diagnostic workup of adults the same is seen in the pediatric settings [38]. This is also important in the treatment monitoring response to show that the inflammation has subsided is there any recurrence or flaring up of the disease.

4.6 Dual Point Imaging in Breast

The role of dual point imaging in breast pathology is to differentiate between focal mastitis, fibroadenoma, and malignant lesion. The important point to be noted here is that breast cancers are small in size and low grade, so it will be difficult to distinguish between these pathologies. This DTPI shows the increased uptake in malignant lesions in comparison with the normal breast parenchyma. Again, it is more helpful in the different settings of delayed imaging to reflect the biology and degree of aggressiveness of the malignant lesions. The principle of dual point delayed imaging is the same. This can be quantified with the SUV max values.

4.7 Limitations of DTPI

There are some limitations of DTPI the important one is to differentiate between the inflammatory and malignant lesions in every setting. The majority of these lesions like lung lesions, lung nodules, mediastinal nodes, granulomatous lesions, and tuberculosis, which are having many overlaps in the DTPI findings. There is also the issue related with the acute, chronic, and acute on chronic inflammatory pathologies which changes the presentations example is acute, chronic, and acute on chronic pancreatitis, this is the result of the Biological behavior of the particular pathology.

4.8 Conclusion

DTPI logically will be able to provide the differentiation between the malignant and the inflammatory pathologies. Thus, it will increase the sensitivity, specificity, and accuracy of FDG PET-CT studies.

References

1. Love C, Tomas MB, Tronco GG, et al. FDG-PET of infection and inflammation. Radiographics. 2005;25:1357–68.
2. Basu S, Alavi A. Unparalleled contribution of ^{18}F-FDG PET to medicine over 3 decades. J Nucl Med. 2008;49:17–21.
3. Zhuang H, Pourdehnad M, Lambright ES, et al. Dual time point ^{18}F-FDG PET imaging for differentiating malignant from inflammatory processes. J Nucl Med. 2001;42:1412–7.
4. Lee ST, Scott AM. Are we ready for dual-time point FDG-PET imaging? J Med Imaging Radiat Oncol. 2011;55:351–2.
5. Basu S, Chryssikos T, Moghadam-Kia S, et al. Positron emission tomography as a diagnostic tool in infection: present role and future possibilities. Semin Nucl Med. 2009;39:36–51.
6. Houshmand S, Salavati A, Basu S, et al. The role of dual and multiple time point imaging of FDG uptake in both normal and disease states. Clin Transl Imaging. 2004;2:281–93.
7. Cheng G, Torigian DA, Zhuang H, et al. When should we recommend use of dual time-point and delayed time-point imaging techniques in FDG PET? Eur J Nucl Med Mol Imaging. 2013;40:779–87.
8. den Hoff J, Hofheinz F, Oehme L, et al. Dual time point based quantification of metabolic uptake rates in 18F-FDG PET. EJNMMI Res. 2013;3:1–6.
9. Chen YM, Huang G, Sun XG, et al. Optimizing delayed scan time for FDG PET: comparison of the early and late delayed scan. Nucl Med Commun. 2008;29:425–30.
10. Hustinx R, Smith RJ, Benard F, et al. Dual time point fluorine-18 fluorodeoxyglucose positron emission tomograpohy: a potential method to differentiate malignancy from inflammation and normal tissue in the head and neck. Eur J Nucl Med. 1999;26:1345–8.
11. Metser U, Even-Sapir E. Increased (18)F-fluorodeoxyglucose uptake in benign, non-physiologic lesions found on whole-body positron emission tomography/computed tomography (PET/CT): accumulated data from four years of experience with PET/CT. Semin Nucl Med. 2007;37:206–22.
12. Lan XL, Zhang YX, Wu ZJ, et al. The value of dual time point (18)F- FDG-PET imaging for the differentiation between malignant and benign lesions. Clin Radiol. 2008;63:756–64.
13. Hamberg LM, Hunter GJ, Alpert NM, et al. The dose uptake eratioasan index of glucose metabolism: useful parameter or oversimplification? J Nucl Med. 1994;35:1308–12.
14. Hustinx R, Smith RJ, Benard F, et al. Dual time point fluorine-18 fluorodeoxyglucose positron emission tomography: a potential method to differentiate malignancy from inflammation and normal tissue in the head and neck. Eur J Nucl Med. 1999;26:1345–8.
15. Farghaly HRS, Sayed MHM, Nasr HA, et al. Dual time point fluorodeoxyglucose positron emission tomography/computed tomography in differentiation between malignant and benign lesions in cancer patients. Does it always work? Indian J Nucl Med. 2015;30:314–9.
16. Gould MK, Maclean CC, Kuschner WG, et al. Accuracy of positron emission tomography for diagnosis of pulmonary nodules and mass lesions: a meta-analysis. JAMA. 2001;21:914–24.
17. Khan AN, Al-Jahdali H. Value of delayed ^{18}F-FDG PET in the diagnosis of solitary pulmonary nodule. J Thorac Dis. 2013;5:373–4.
18. Alkhawaldeh K, Bural G, Kumar R, et al. Impact of dual time point ^{18}F-FDG PET imaging and partial volume correction in the assessment of solitary pulmonary nodules. Eur J Nucl Med Mol Imaging. 2008;35:246–52.
19. Huang YE, Huang YJ, Ko M, et al. Dual-time-point ^{18}F-FDG PET/CT in the diagnosis of solitary pulmonary lesions in a region with endemic granulomatous diseases. Ann Nucl Med. 2016;30:652–8.
20. MacDonald K, Searle J, Lyburn I. The role of dual time point FDG-PET imaging in the evaluation of solitary pulmonary nodules with an initial standard uptake value less than 2.5. Clin Radiol. 2011;66:244–50.
21. Lin YY, Chen JH, Ding HJ, Liang JA, Yeh JJ, Kao CH. Potential value of dual-time-point (1) (8)F-FDG PET compared with initial single-time-point imaging in differentiating malignant

from benign pulmonary nodules: a systematic review and meta-analysis. Nucl Med Commun. 2012;33(10):1011–8.

22. Suga K, Kawakami Y, Hiyama A, et al. Dual-time point 18F-FDG- PET/CT scan for differentiation between 18F-FDG avid non-small cell lung cancer and benign lesions. Ann Nucl Med. 2009;23:427–35.

23. Feldman F, Jeerti RV, Manos C. ^{18}F-FDG PET scanning of benign and malignant musculoskeletal lesions. Skelet Radiol. 2003;32:201–8.

24. Lan XL, Zhang YX, Wu ZJ, et al. The value of dual time point ^{18}F-FDG PET imaging for the differentiation between malignant and benign lesions. Clin Radiol. 2008;63:756–64.

25. Hong SP, Lee SE, Choi YL, et al. Prognostic value of 18F-FDG PET/CT in patients with soft tissue sarcoma: comparisons between metabolic parameters. Skelet Radiol. 2014;43:641–8.

26. Shin DS, Shon OJ, Han DS, et al. The clinical efficacy of 18F-FDG PET/CT in benign and malignant musculoskeletal tumors. Ann Nucl Med. 2008;22:603–9.

27. Sahlmann CO, Siefker U, Lehmann K, et al. Dual time point 2 ^{18}F fluoro-2' deoxyglucose positron emission tomograpohy in chronic bacterial osteomyelitis. Nucl Med Commun. 2004;25:819–23.

28. Tian R, Su M, Tian Y, et al. Dual time point PET-CT with F-18 FDG forth differentiation of malignant and benign bone lesions. Skelet Radiol. 2009;38:451/458.

29. Dirisamer A, Halpern BS, Schima W, et al. Dual time point FDG PET-CT forth detection of hepatic metastases. Mol Imaging Biol. 2008;10:335–40.

30. Arena V, Skanjeti A, Casoni R, et al. Dual-phase FDG-PET: delayed acquisition improves hepatic detectability of pathological uptake. Radiol Med. 2008;113:875–86.

31. Nishiyama Y, Yamamoto Y, Fukunaga K, et al. Dual-time-point 18F-FDG-PET for the evaluation of gallbladder carcinoma. J Nucl Med. 2006;47:633–8.

32. Lyshchik A, Higashi T, Nakamoto Y, et al. Dual-phase 18F-fluoro-2- deoxy-D-glucose positron emission tomography as a prognostic parameter in patients with pancreatic cancer. Eur J Nucl Med Mol Imaging. 2005;32:389–97.

33. Higashi T, Saga T, Nakamoto Y, et al. Relationship between retention index in dual-phase (18) F-FDG-PET, and hexokinase-II and glucosetransporter-1 expression in pancreatic cancer. J Nucl Med. 2002;43:173–80.

34. Nakamoto Y, Higashi T, Sakahara H, et al. Delayed (18)F-fluoro-2-deoxy-D-glucose positron emission tomography scan for differentiation between malignant and benign lesions in the pancreas. Cancer. 2000;89:2547–54.

35. Metser U, Miller E, Kessler A, Lerman H, Lievshitz G, Oren R, et al. Solid splenic masses: evaluation with FFDG PET/CT. J Nucl Med. 2005;46:52–9.

36. Vaidyanathan S, Patel CN, Scarsbrook AF, Chowdhury FU. FDG PET/CT in infection and inflammation–current and emerging clinical applications. Clin Radiol. 2015;70:787–800. https://doi.org/10.1016/j.crad.2015.03.010.

37. Van Limbergen J, Russell RK, Drummond HE, Aldhous MC, Round NK, Nimmo ER, Smith L, Gillett PM, McGrogan P, Weaver LT, Bisset WM, Mahdi G, Arnott ID, Satsangi J, Wilson DC. Definition of phenotypic characteristics of childhood-onset inflammatory bowel disease. Gastroenterology. 2008;135:1114–22.

38. Mavi A, Urhan M, Yu JQ, et al. Dual time point 18F-FDG-PET imaging detects breast cancer with high sensitivity and correlates well with histologic subtypes. J Nucl Med. 2006;47:1440–6.

PET-CT in Fever of Unknown Origin

5

Key Points
Fever is an important clinical condition, which is associated with multiple causes. It is diagnosed on basis of presenting symptoms, physical examination, and routine investigations of blood and urine. Despite the large spectrum of causes involved and the variabilities in the clinical aspect it is not precisely diagnosed correctly till date. Many studies and parameters are involved in this evaluation but not a single modality or specialty could define this and diagnose it. Fever is associated with various systems involvement presenting with various system-specific clinical findings [1–4]. Many routines and conventional imaging modalities are available for the diagnosis with varying results, sensitivity, and specificity. FDG PET-CT has evolved in many aspects to diagnose more precisely of various pathologies [5, 6]. The commonest use of the FDG PET-CT is for malignancy and is now followed by the evalaution of the various nonmalignant conditions. The Nonmalignant conditions play an important component where FDG PET-CT has evolved, In this category, infection and inflammation are the most important and commonest indications with varieties of causes like Bacterial, Viral, Fungal, and other associated pathologies.

5.1 Introduction

5.1.1 Fever of Unknown Origin

Fever of Unknown Origin (FUO) is defined as the recurrent fever of 38.3 °C or higher, lasting 2–3 weeks or longer and undiagnosed after 1 week of hospital evaluation. The three most important causes of FUO are Infections, Malignancies, and Nonmalignant Inflammatory conditions. The systematic approach for diagnosis of FUO, which is followed are physical examination, various laboratory investigations, simple interventional procedures, and various imaging modalities. The first and foremost line of evaluation of FUO depend on the facilities and expertise

© The Author(s), under exclusive license to Springer Nature
Singapore Pte Ltd. 2021
S. Shaikh, *PET-CT in Infection and Inflammation*,
https://doi.org/10.1007/978-981-15-9801-2_5

available at that time and region. Most of the time the evaluation starts with step-by-step approach using different available modes of investigation. Usually, the higher modalities of the evaluation come in a later stage when the primary and common investigations are either normal or not confirmative or need higher evaluation. In this scenario, the role of PET-CT in FUO is debatable where usually it is not advised as the first line of investigation. However, at some places and in our institute PET-CT is advised if it fits clearly in the criteria and definition of FUO. The biggest advantage of PET-CT is to identify the cause of FUO in form of infective focus and second will be other associated organs or system involvement, this we can do at one time. Thus, saving time and other unwarranted investigations. The basic concept of the PET-CT is the glucose metabolism which is related to GLUT metabolism due to overproduction of the glycolytic enzymes. In the major studies, the diagnosis of infection and inflammation by the PET-CT scan is approx. 25–60% [7, 8].

5.1.2   Imaging Modalities in the Evaluation of FUO

Routine conventional imaging modalities like Radiographs, Ultrasound, Color Doppler, CT, MRI, and Interventional Radiology are being widely used in the evaluation of FUO to rule out possibilities like mass lesions, malignancies, and abscesses. Nuclear Medicine studies like Radionuclide studies allow the detection of possible focus causing the FUO but sensitivity of radionuclide studies is not high compared to anatomical modalities. With this radiolabeled WBC and Ga67-citrate are used to evaluate the acute, chronic, granulomatous, and autoimmune infections, inflammations, and malignant diseases [9, 10]. With the advent of FDG PET-CT, the radionuclide imaging is not being widely used. FDG has shown a significant range of accuracy. In a prospective study involving 74 patients, Buysschaert and colleagues [11] found that FDG PET is extremely sensitive in diagnosis. A recent study has concluded that the accuracy of FDG PET-CT in FUO is better compared to routine CT and other imaging modalities.

5.1.3   FDG PET-CT in Evaluation of FUO

Infection is the most common cause of FUO in children [12]. This is also very common in the adult age groups. Inflammatory diseases rank second after infection as a cause of FUO in pediatric patients. Various conditions in this pediatrics age group are autoimmune, connective tissue, vasculitis, granulomatous disorders, endocrine disorders, and subacute thyroiditis.

5.1.4   Glucose Metabolism

Three mechanisms of Glucose transport are responsible for (1) 18F FDG metabolism, (2) passive diffusion, active transport GLUT, and (3) transporting to human cells GLUT1 and GLUT13. Biodistribution of 18F FDG is preferably taken up in tissues with high glucose consumption. Excretion is done by the kidney [13].

Uptake in inflammatory cells is by lymphocytes which are activated and show an increased uptake on 18FDG and this FDG uptake is directly proportional to the infective inflammatory activity.

5.1.5 Various Conditions of FUO

There are multiple causes of FUO comprising traumatic, infective inflammatory, malignant, and metabolic miscellaneous causes. The majority of this is comprised of infective inflammatory pathologies. The various causes may involve the single system, or multiple systems or may involve all systems involving the central nervous system, head and neck, respiratory, cardiac, GIT, GUT, musculoskeletal, and miscellaneous causes [14–20]. Depending on the system involvement, the morbidity of the patient can be defined. FDG PET-CT has become an ideal tool for identifying and diagnosing the focus of infection and to identify the relapse of the infections in relation to the therapy response. The response to the therapy is associated with partial response, complete response, and disease progression. This FDG PET-CT also plays an important role in the evaluation of critically ill patients who are suspected of infection and cannot be mobilized for multiple investigations at multiple times. Another major cause of FUO is malignant conditions and also with associated superadded infection along with malignancy, during the treatment, or as a complication to the treatment. In a study involving 33 patients in the ICU, Simon and colleagues [21] found that PET-CT has a sensitivity of 100% and specificity of 79% in identifying the source of infection. The exact experience on the role of FDG PET-CT in the evaluation of FUO in the pediatric population is still limited and lot more to be done for making specific protocols. One of the commonest reasons is not much advised due to radiation and ALARA aspects. A couple of studies has shown that FDG PET-CT is very important with the management of pediatric patients suffering from FUO. In one of the large multicentric studies involving pediatric patients (569) using FDG PET-CT the diagnosis of FUO was established in 73% of patients. Here, the disadvantages of using PET-CT for pediatric age groups are radiation dose which has to be meticulously planned to reduce the radiation dose. One of the studies by Ferda and colleagues [22] who used this approach evaluated 48 patients of FUO and was able to diagnose fever in 43 patients. Some investigators believe that the use of FDG PET-CT has to be used only in adult patients with FUO and with elevated parameters of raised ESR and C-reactive protein [23]. FDG PET-CT here is important in detecting the early focus of infection or inflammation. With newer techniques in the PET-CT and new radiotracers, PET-CT is evolving more and more with higher sensitivities and will be more useful in further diagnosing more and newer infective inflammatory conditions. Thus, normal FDG PET-CT excludes the probable infective cause in the majority of cases and helps in ruling out the active focus of infection or inflammation (Figs. 5.1, 5.2, 5.3, 5.4, 5.5, 5.6, 5.7, 5.8, 5.9 and 5.10).

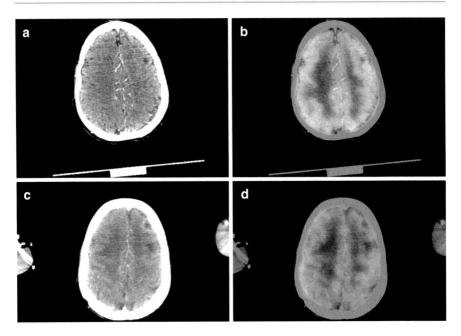

Fig. 5.1 Limited brain PET-CT, CT image (**a**) and (**c**) showing mild meningeal enhancement in the left frontoparietal region with no significant increase in the tracer activity on (**b**) and (**d**) images. FDG radiotracer for brain lesions is not sensitive. This patient with FUO was diagnosed as meningitis

5.1.6 Advantages of FDG PET-CT Over Conventional Radionuclide Studies in Infection and Inflammation

- High sensitivity.
- High resolution images.
- High target-to-background ratio.
- Fast technique completed in one session (Fig. 5.10).

The advantages of over other modalities are also there as single modality with single scan can give more precise information. The only difference will be the lesser soft tissue sensitivities as compared to MRI. However, PET-MR will be more useful and give better answers for most of the soft tissues involved and especially pediatric patients (Figs. 5.11, 5.12, 5.13, 5.14, 5.15, 5.16, 5.17, and 5.18).

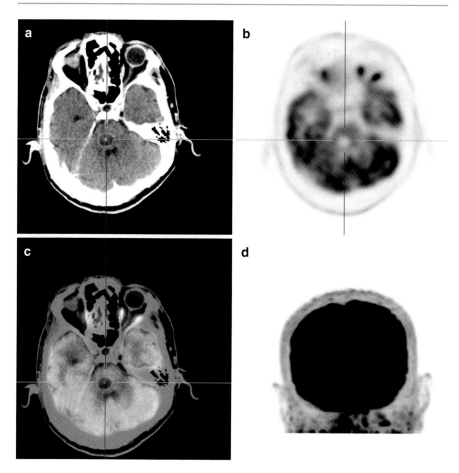

Fig. 5.2   Brain PET-CT, CT image (**a**) showing ring-enhancing lesion with a tiny enhancing mural nodule in the pons suggestive of neurocysticercosis. PET images (**b**) and (**d**) showing no tracer activity and fuse image (**c**) showing no significant tracer activity. This patient presented with FUO

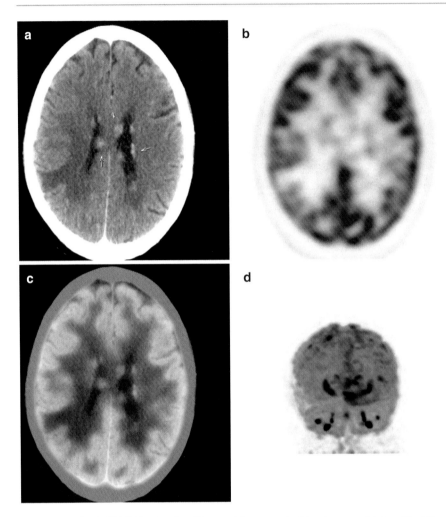

Fig. 5.3 Limited PET-CT brain of an 25-year old presented with seizures and intermittent fever under the FUO. CT image (**a**) showing small irregular enhancing subependymal nodules suggestive of tuberous sclerosis. No abnormal uptake noted in this corresponding nodule in PET images (**b**) and (**d**) and fused (**c**) image. Tuberous sclerosis also presents FUO

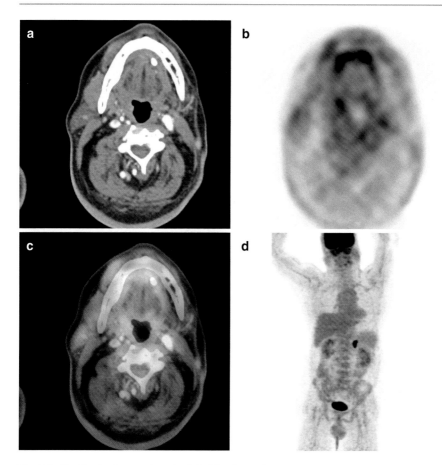

Fig. 5.4 Small calculus noted on the left side of mandible in CT image (**a**) with associated mild FDG uptake in fused (**c**) image and (**b**) and (**d**) PET images suggestive of sialolith involving sublingual gland

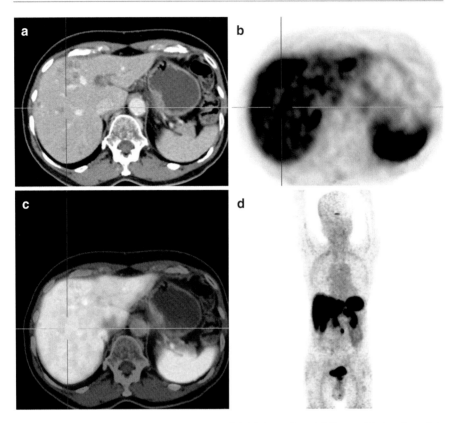

Fig. 5.5 A 32-year old with FUO. Whole-body PET-CT was done, CT image (**a**) showing subtle irregular hypodense lesions noted involving the right lobe of the liver. Diffuse increased uptake noted in the entire liver parenchyma in PET images (**b**) and (**d**) and fused image (**c**). Rest of the whole body appears normal. Findings are consistent with Hepatitis and this was Hepatitis B

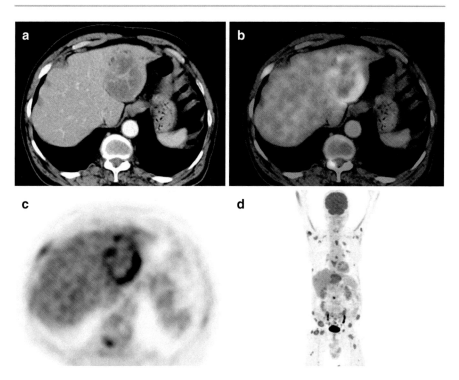

Fig. 5.6 Whole-body PET showing multiple metabolically active lesions involving the bones from a multiple myeloma patient of known case. Incidentally, a hypodense patchily enhancing lesion in left lobe of the liver in CT images (**a**) consistent with Hydatic cyst, and fused image (**b**) and PET images (**c**) and (**d**) shows minimal uptake in the periphery of this lesion, post-operatively confirmed by histopathology

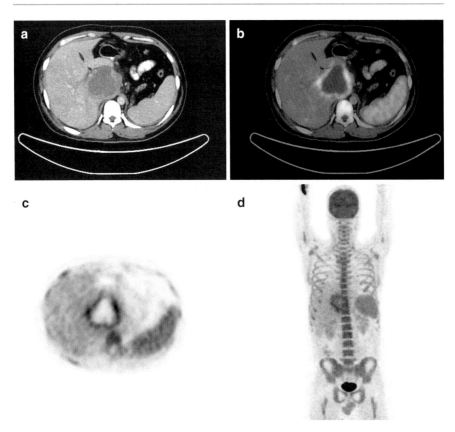

Fig. 5.7 (**a**) CT showing hypodense lesion with patchy wall enhancement in segment-I of the liver, (**b**) with SUV max of 3.5 suggestive of liver abscess, Irregular mild uptake seen in the PET (**c**) and fused images, (**d**) A 48-year old with FUO. Whole-body PET-CT

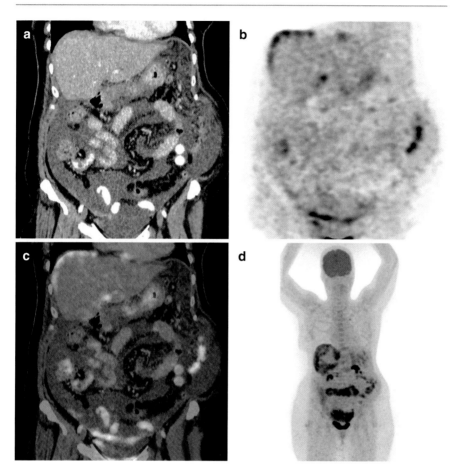

Fig. 5.8 A 51-year female with FUO and abdominal pain on and off for 1 month. Loss of weight and loss of appetite. Whole-body PET-CT showing diffuse irregular peritoneal thickening with small nodularity and associated mild-to-moderate ascites on CT image (**a**) and mild uptake in the peritoneal nodule with SUV max of 4.8 on PET (**b**). (**d**) and PET-CT images (**c**). Features are suggestive of peritonitis

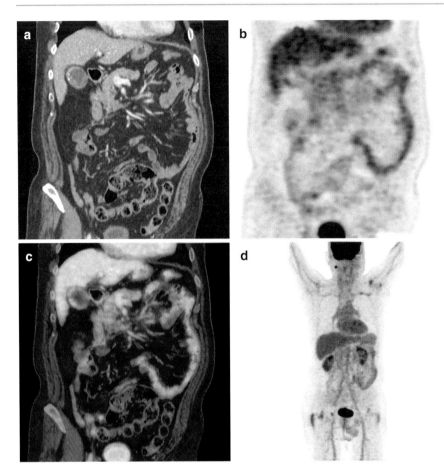

Fig. 5.9 A 42-year old presenting with right hypochondriac pain with clinical Murphy's sign positive and FUO for the last 1 month. PET-CT findings show tiny gall bladder calculi with sludge and associated focal wall thickening in the fundus (**a**) with associated focal mild metabolic activity SUV max of 3.5 (**b**), (**c**) and (**d**) suggestive of calculous cholecystitis

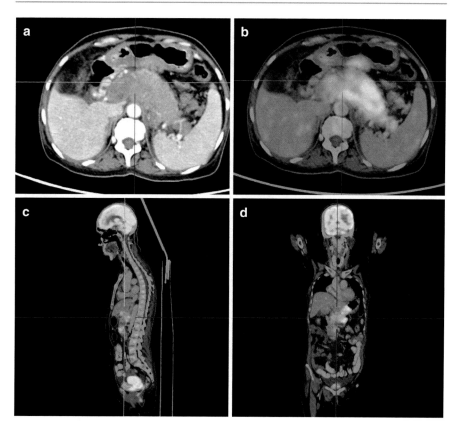

Fig. 5.10 A 39-year-old male with severe epigastric pain for the last 2 days, more severe in the last 6 h with episodes of continuous vomiting and FUO. Whole-body PET-CT, CT showing diffusely bulky pancreas (**a**) with fused PET-CT images (**b**), (**c**) and (**d**) showing diffusely increased uptake SUV max of 8.2 and effacement of peripancreatic fat plane suggestive of acute pancreatitis

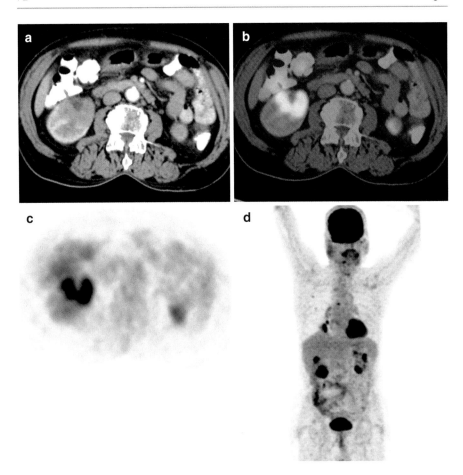

Fig. 5.11 History of FUO with cough and expectoration. Chest radiograph showing right lower lobe patchy pneumonitis. Whole-body PET-CT under FUO protocol, CT image (**a**) reveals irregular hypodense non-enhancing areas in both kidneys, largest seen in lower pole of right kidney suggestive of acute pyelonephritis. Corresponding fused PET-CT image (**b**) and PET images (**c**) and (**d**) showing focal uptake with SUV max of 5.2

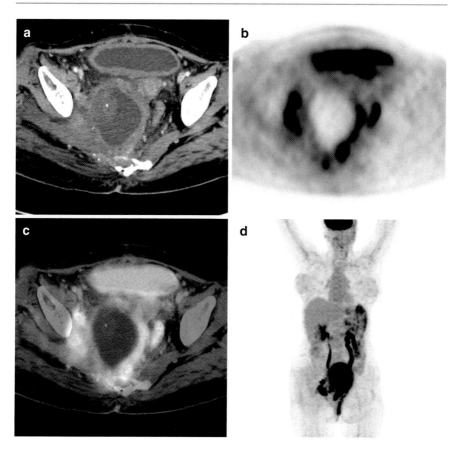

Fig. 5.12 Status post-hysterectomy. FUO post-surgery, severe pain in lower abdomen, and constipation on and off. Whole-body PET-CT, CT image (**a**) showing an irregular thick-walled collection in right lower pelvis involving the right pelvic floor muscles and PET (**b**), (**d**) and fused PET-CT images (**c**) showing peripheral wall enhancement of this collection with SUV max of 6.7

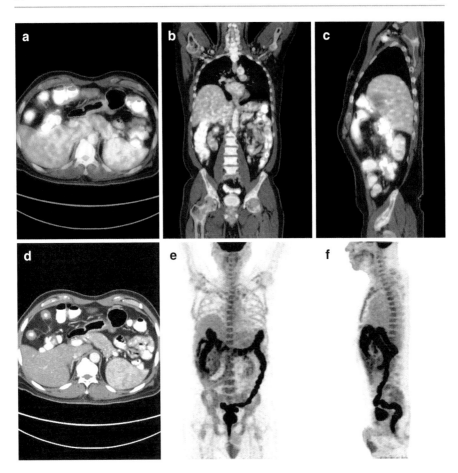

Fig. 5.13 A 52-year-old male with intermittent diarrhea and constipation and loss of weight with FUO. Whole-body PET-CT, CT image (**a**) showing diffuse irregular circumferential wall thickening involving the ascending colon and hepatic flexure with significant narrowing of the lumen and fused PET-CT (**a**), (**b**), (**c**) and PET images (**e**) and (**f**) show subtle mild uptake, this cannot be differentiated clearly due to physiological bowel uptake. Findings are suggestive of Crohn's disease

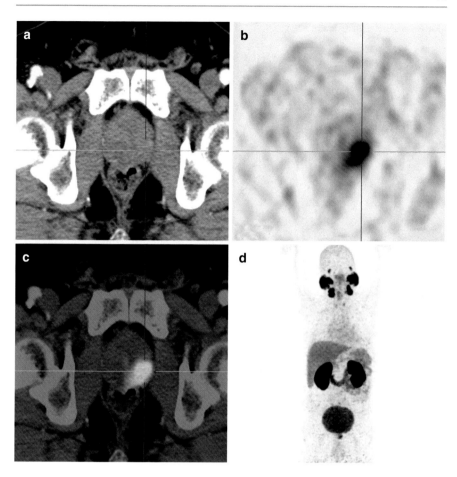

Fig. 5.14 FUO with burning micturition for 3 weeks, borderline PSA of 5. Whole-body PET-CT with PSMA was done, CT image (**a**) was normal and fused PET-CT images (**b**), (**c**), and (**d**) showing the focal area of increased uptake in the left lateral lobe of prostate. Possibility of malignancy was suspected with SUV max of 8.2. However, TRUS biopsy showed a focal area of prostatitis

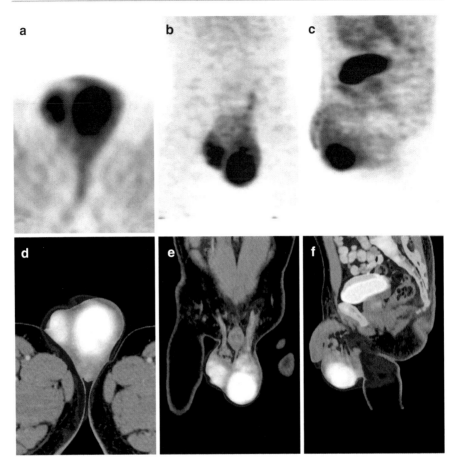

Fig. 5.15 Testicular pain on and off with fever. Limited pelvis PET-CT showing diffuse increased FDG uptake with SUV max of 10 in PET images (**a**), (**b**), and (**c**) and fused PET-CT images (**d**), (**e**), and (**f**). Findings suggestive of diffuse orchitis left testes

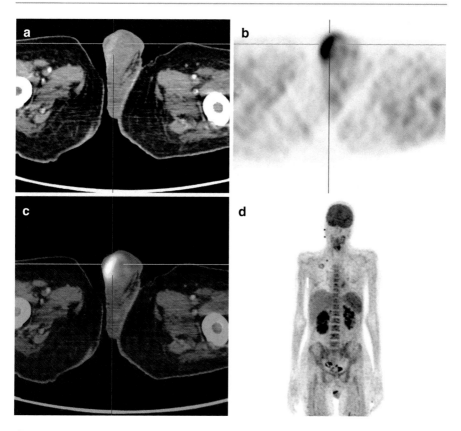

Fig. 5.16 Mild fever on and off with FUO. Mild tenderness on right side of the scrotum. Whole-body PET-CT done under FUO protocol showing mild heterogenous enhancement on CT image (**a**) and shows diffuse increased uptake on PET (**b**) (**d**) and fused PET-CT images (**c**) with SUV max of 7.1 involving right scrotal wall suggestive of scrotal wall inflammatory changes

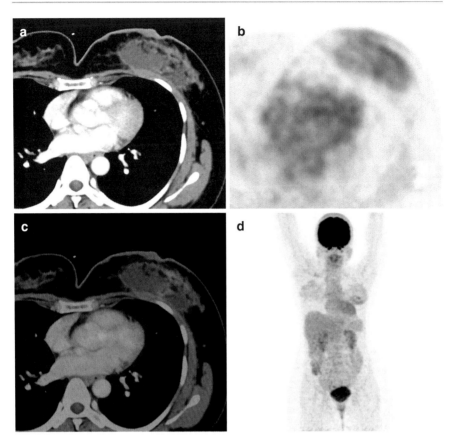

Fig. 5.17 Mild fever with tenderness left breast parenchyma for 1 month. Whole PET-CT evaluated showing mild patchy enhancement on CT image (**a**) with minimal FDG uptake with SUV max of 2.1 on PET-CT and PET images (**b**), (**c**), and (**d**). In addition, CT showing small areas of loculated fluid collection suggestive of mastitis

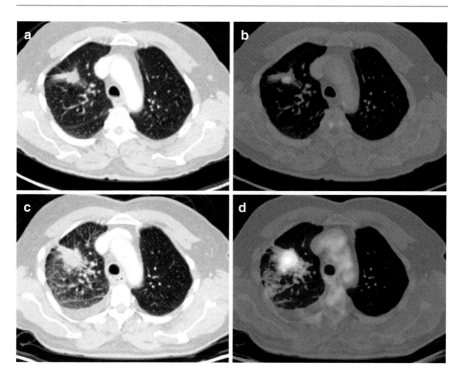

Fig. 5.18 FUO advised whole-body PET-CT, CT images (**a**) and (**c**) showing irregular parenchymal nodular lesion with increased uptake with SUV max of 6.2 seen on fused images (**b**) and (**d**) and adjacent fibrotic strands, focal pleural thickening and parenchymal infiltrates. Findings are suggestive of pulmonary Koch's

5.2   Summary

FUO is an important and sometimes complex entity, which can be diagnosed by FDG PET-CT in a very early stage helping in very early diagnosis and reducing the morbidity and hospitalization and unnecessary tests. There are many important causes of FUO, which will be discussed in the coming chapters. Thus, the PET-CT is an ideal investigation, which will potentially replace all other imaging modalities by virtue of its better diagnostic capabilities, higher sensitivity, and a wide spectrum of diseases to be analyzed. Thus, FDG PET-CT is an important diagnostic modality due to the wider applications and higher sensitivities.

References

1. de Kleijn EM, van Lier HJ, van der Meer JW. Fever of unknown origin (FUO). II. Diagnostic procedures in a prospective multicenter study of 167 patients. The Netherlands FUO Study Group. Medicine (Baltimore). 1997;76:401–14.
2. Bleeker-Rovers CP, Vos FJ, de Kleijn EM, et al. A prospective multicenter study on fever of unknown origin: the yield of a structured diagnostic protocol. Medicine (Baltimore). 2007;86:26–38.
3. Vanderschueren S, Del Biondo E, Ruttens D, et al. Inflammation of unknown origin versus fever of unknown origin: two of a kind. Eur J Intern Med. 2009;20:415–8.
4. Vanderschueren S, Knockaert D, Adriaenssens T, et al. From prolonged febrile illness to fever of unknown origin: the challenge continues. Arch Intern Med. 2003;163:1033–41.
5. Blockmans D, Knockaert D, Maes A, et al. Clinical value of [(18)F]fluorodeoxyglucose positron emission tomography for patients with fever of unknown origin. Clin Infect Dis. 2001;32:191–6.
6. Lorenzen J, Buchert R, Bohuslavizki KH. Value of FDG PET in patients with fever of unknown origin. Nucl Med Commun. 2001;22:779–83.
7. Meller J, Altenvoerde G, Munzel U, et al. Fever of unknown origin: prospective comparison of [18F]FDG imaging with a double-head coincidence camera and gallium-67 citrate SPET. Eur J Nucl Med. 2000;27:1617–25.
8. Bleeker-Rovers CP, de Kleijn EM, Corstens FH, et al. Clinical value of FDG PET in patients with fever of unknown origin and patients suspected of focal infection or inflammation. Eur J Nucl Med Mol Imaging. 2004;31:29–37.
9. Signore A, Glaudemans AWJM, Malviya G, Lazzeri E, Prandini N, Viglietti AL, et al. Development and testing of a new disposable sterile device for labelling white blood cells. Q J Nucl Med Mol Imaging. 2012;56(4):400–8.
10. Wang L, Yang H, Zhao X, Cai J, Zhu Z, Li F. Feasibility of 18F-FDG combination with 68Ga-citrate PET/CT in the diagnosis of inflammatory bowel disease—first results. J Nucl Med. 2014;55:381.
11. Buysschaert I, Vanderschueren S, Blockmans D, Mortelmans L, Knockaert D. Contribution of (18) fluoro-deoxyglucose positron emission tomography to the work-up of patients with fever of un- knownorigin. Eur J Intern Med. 2004;15:151–6.
12. Chang L, Cheng MF, Jou ST, et al. Search of unknown fever focus using PET in critically ill children with complicated underlying diseases. Pediatr Crit Care Med. 2016;17:e58–65.
13. Scholtens AM, Verberne HJ, Budde RP, et al. Additional heparin pre-administration improves cardiac glucose metabolism suppression over low-carbohydrate diet alone in (1)(8)F-FDG PET imaging. J Nucl Med. 2016;57:568–73.

14. Semmler A, Hermann S, Mormann F, Weberpals M, Paxian SA, Okulla T, et al. Sepsis causes neuro-inflammation and concomitant decrease of cerebral metabolism. J Neuroinflammation. 2008;5:38.
15. Balink H, Verberne HJ, Bennink RJ, et al. A rationale for the use of F18-FDG PET/CT in fever and inflammation of unknown origin. Int J Mol Imaging. 2012;2012:165080.
16. Federici L, Blondet C, Imperiale A, Sibilia J, Pasquali JL, Pflumio F, et al. Value of (18) F-FDG-PET/CT in patients with fever of unknown origin and unexplained prolonged inflammatory syndrome: a single centre analysis experience. Int J Clin Pract. 2010;64:55–60.
17. Habib G, Lancellotti P, Antunes MJ, Bongiorni MG, Casalta JP, Del Zotti FESC, et al. ESC 2015 guidelines on management of infective endocarditis. Eur Heart J. 2015;36:3075–128.
18. Vaidyanathan S, Patel CN, Scarsbrook AF, Chowdhury FU. FDG PET/CT in infection and inflammation—current and emerging clinical applications. Clin Radiol. 2015;70:787–800.
19. van der Bruggen W, Bleeker-Rovers CP, Boerman OC, et al. PET and SPECT in osteomyelitis and prosthetic bone and joint infections: a systematic review. Semin Nucl Med. 2010;40:3–15.
20. Martin C, Castaigne C, Tondeur M, et al. Role and interpretation of fluorodeoxyglucose-positron emission tomography/computed tomography in HIV-infected patients with fever of unknown origin: a prospective study. HIV Med. 2013;14:455–62.
21. Mulders-Manders C, Simon A, Bleeker-Rovers C. Fever of unknown origin. Clin Med (Lond). 2015;15:280–4.
22. Ferda J, Ferdova E, Zahlava J, et al. Fever of unknown origin: a value of (18)F-FDG-PET/CT with integrated full diagnostic isotropic CT imaging. Eur J Radiol. 2010;73:518–25.
23. Balink H, Veeger NJ, Bennink RJ, et al. The predictive value of C-reactive protein and erythrocyte sedimentation rate for 18F-FDG PET/CT outcome in patients with fever and inflammation of unknown origin. Nucl Med Commun. 2015;36:604–9.

PET-CT in Chest Infective Inflammatory Pathologies

6

Key Points

PET-CT is the hybrid imaging modality, which is a well-established diagnostic imaging modality for Oncological Pathologies and with the advent of the newer radiotracers and advancements in the PET-CT and in the radiotracers newer applications are seen in the form of infection and inflammation. 18 FDG is the most widely used radiotracer, which demonstrates the metabolic activity in various tissues. In these inflammatory cells are activated which metabolites the glucose as source of energy and with this concept FDG is being used to detect various infective and inflammatory conditions and many newer pathologies an be evaluated.

6.1   Introduction

PET-CT is a well-established imaging modality and has the capacity to image the labelled compounds in the body [1]. With the same principle of FDG uptake, various nonmalignant conditions can be evaluated like lung, pleura, and mediastinal lesions. In the infective and inflammatory pathologies chain of reactions happen due to release of the various local factor's cytokines, interleukins, and prostaglandins [2, 3]. These pro-inflammatory mediators regulate the cascade of reactions with migration of the neutrophils, monocytes, and mast cells. The inflammatory response is mediated and facilitating glucose metabolism [4]. With this accumulation of all these cells and increased capillary permeability in the infection the inflammatory cells like granulocytes, leukocytes, and macrophages. This is the basis of the FDG uptake in the infective and inflammatory lesions [5].

PET-CT shows diffuse increased uptake secondary to the glucose metabolism triggered by various cascades of the inflammatory reactions. This increased FDG uptake is also dependent on the neutrophil activity, which takes the FDG uptake due to the activation of the pulmonary alveolar and interstitial macrophages [6].

© The Author(s), under exclusive license to Springer Nature
Singapore Pte Ltd. 2021
S. Shaikh, *PET-CT in Infection and Inflammation*,
https://doi.org/10.1007/978-981-15-9801-2_6

FDG PET-CT has an important role in the evaluation of various pulmonary and extrapulmonary lesions. PET-CT helps to differentiate benign and malignant lesions. Recent technical advancements in PET-CT have increased the barrier of diagnostic work-up of various chest pathologies.

With this 18F FDG PET-CT is the important imaging modality, which has shown a significant increase in accuracy, advantage of noninvasive imaging modality, and most important differentiating between benign and malignant pulmonary lesions. Some benign lesions may appear as false positive and or non-specific. The objective of this study is to characterize the different pulmonary lesions, pleural lesions, and associated systemic pathology, which involve the pulmonary, pleural, and other chest lesions [7]. Thus, plays an important role in the differential diagnosis of benign pulmonary lesions.

6.2   PET-CT Acquisition

6.2.1   Acquisition Protocol

18F FDG PET-CT images were obtained using the Somaton Siemens biograph PET-CT machine with 16 slice CT scanner and high-resolution PET component [8]. All patients were injected with 18F FDG 1 h before the examination as per the weight and patient requirement. A contrast whole-body CT scan was done followed by PET. Delayed PET-CT scans were taken wherever required depending on the patient basis. A dedicated lung window was also acquired in the full inspiratory phase (Fig. 6.1).

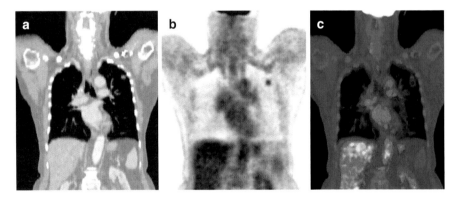

Fig. 6.1 Limited PET-CT chest showing tiny nodule in the left upper lobe. This nodule in CT image (**a**), PET image (**b**), and fused image (**c**). The fused image shows misregistration of this nodule due to technical aspect. CT taken in full inspiration and PET done in normal breathing. Sometimes this will appear as there are two nodules

6.2.2   Image Analysis

The quantification of 18F FDG PET is based on the semiquantitative analysis measured by standardized SUV max values. The usual method of quantification is to set the ROI at the location of lung lesions. With the modern PET-CT systems, this SUV max can be quantified automatically. The anatomical measurements can be done routinely.

6.3   Lung Lesions

6.3.1   Primary Lung Lesions

PET-CT has evolved as an important imaging modality with the rapid development of structural and functional components. With the extensive use of PET in the oncological settings, a lot of concurrent nonmalignant lesions were also evaluated with different imaging parameters and characteristics. This has led to a keen interest in the evaluation of nonmalignant lesions. Initially, it was difficult and had to be confirmed by histopathology. But now with newer imaging techniques and protocols, it has become easier to distinguish between benign and malignant lesions and infective inflammatory and malignant lesions. With this scenario, many PET-CT scans are being advised for evaluation of various infective inflammatory, granulomatous, and benign pathologies of the lung. Various lung pathologies which are affected in various infective inflammatory pathologies and can be evaluated. The varied presentations of lung pathologies are solitary pulmonary nodule, patchy infiltrates, patchy parenchymal nodules, cavitary lesions, ground glass opacities, alveolar opacities, interstitial lesions, reticulonodular lesions, interstitial thickening, mass lesion with or without collapse consolidation, and combination of the components mentioned above [5, 9]. The malignant pathologies also most of the times have similar presentations that can be difficult to differentiate between malignant and nonmalignant entities. Other lesions like granulomatous, metabolic, and sometimes traumatic and most important tuberculosis also have to be ruled out or confirmed [10–14]. With the SUV max quantification, it is difficult to distinguish between the two, especially when there is no significant difference or disparity in the clinical findings between the two (Figs. 6.2, 6.3, 6.4, and 6.5).

Larger lesions cavitation's, patchy consolidations involving a segment or extending into another segment which can be evaluated further, and the differentials will depend on the clinical settings can be tuberculosis or malignant lesions or collagen granulomas. The alveolar and ground glass opacities are mostly related to the perilesional component [15]. However, exclusive alveolar opacities can be seen in bronchoalveolar carcinomas [16], which have to be differentiated between the two (Figs. 6.6, 6.7, and 6.8).

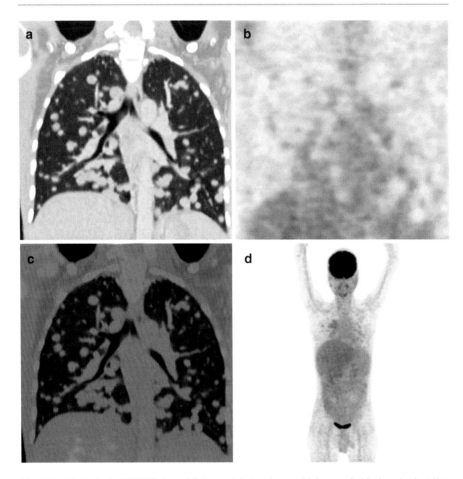

Fig. 6.2 Whole-body PET-CT done CT image (**a**) showing multiple rounded lesions in the bilateral lung parenchyma. PET (**b, d**) and fused PET-CT images (**c**) showing multiple nodular lesions in both lungs with no FDG activity suggestive of multiple inactive granulomas

6.3.2   Protocol of Evaluation

The newer protocol for the evaluation is dual time point imaging. Here, the delayed PET is done after 1 h of the primary PET scan or it can be after 2 or 3 h of the primary PET scan. The concept of this delayed scan is the metabolically active tracer activity is dependent on the malignant potential in which the radiotracer will be retained in delayed scan causing SUV max to be static. However, in nonmalignant, infective inflammatory, and other benign entities, the SUV max in the region of interest significantly reduces compared to the primary PET scan [17]. However, this does not apply in all cases. However, with this protocol a lot of fallacies are there.

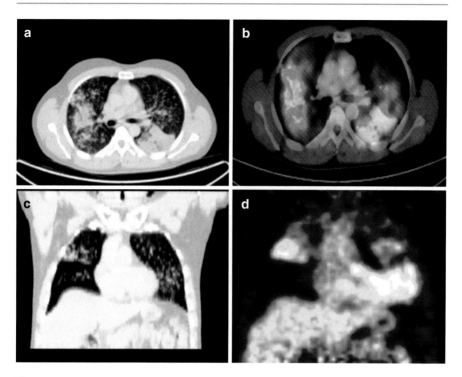

Fig. 6.3 Limited PET-CT chest done showing bronchioalveolar opacity in both lungs with associated tiny nodular opacities (**a, c**) with increased FDG uptake in PET-CT (**b**) and PET-CT (**d**) both
lungs of SUV max of 4.5 suggestive of bronchioalveolar pathology. Histopathology confirmed
consolidation

The other infective inflammatory conditions of the chest are fungal lesions,
granulomatous infections, fibrosing mediastinitis, organizing pneumonia, granulomatosis with polyangiitis, and histiocytic processes like Erdheim-chester disease. One of another important indications is to monitor the lesions or disease
after the treatment. If there is an infective inflammatory cavitatory lesion, then
can be evaluated after the antibiotic therapy [18]. But this is not routinely used
protocol for post-therapy evaluation in infective inflammatory pathologies as this
can be done easily with the routine conventional imaging modalities like radiographs, CT chest, or MRI. Sometimes, it is difficult to evaluate the associated
concurrent infective inflammatory lesions in malignant settings or immunocompromised status of a patient or it can be a superadded infection, which is secondary to the malignant therapy complications. Here, PET-CT has a significant role
because the metabolic activity there is in the primary lesion and adjacent secondary lesion. Other than FDG PET newer radiotracers are in pipeline for the
evaluation.

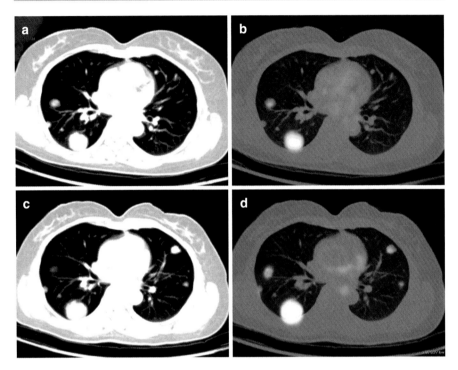

Fig. 6.4 Whole-body PET-CT at the level of chest showing multiple nodular lesions (**a**, **c**) with significant metabolic activity in PET-CT (**b**, **d**) with largest one in right lower lobe with SUV max of 8.9 suggestive of active granulomas. Rest of the whole body appears normal

6.3.3   Noninfectious Lung Lesions

PET-CT is also helpful in the evaluation of the many noninfectious lung diseases like COPD, Asthma, Pneumoconiosis, Sarcoidosis, and many miscellaneous conditions.

COPD is chronic obstructive pulmonary disease due to Smoking or Asthma. One of the important aspects is to differentiate COPD due to Smoking and Asthma, the criteria here is inflammation in the smoking, which will show increased uptake [19, 20]. Another aspect is the respiratory muscle uptake due to increased effort for respiration. To quantify the respiratory muscle uptake, which shows the efforts in respiration and to diagnose the complication of COPD like corpulmonale.

6.3.4   Pneumoconiosis

Pneumoconiosis is the parenchymal reaction to the inhalation of the toxic materials for those working in occupational exposure. A good deal of Pneumoconiosis like Coal workers, silicosis, Asbestosis, and Berylliosis. Here the inhalation of the toxic dust will cause the inflammatory reaction that progresses to the loss of function and

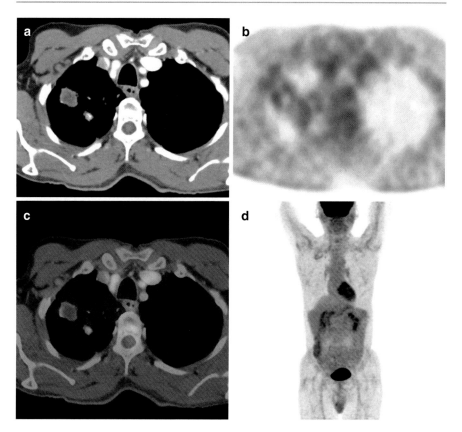

Fig. 6.5 Whole-body PET-CT showing a small nodular lesion in the right upper lobe of the lung (**a**) with minimal uptake (**b–d**) with SUV max of 1.8 suggestive of benign solitary pulmonary nodule

permanent scarring. Here the PET-CT plays an important role in monitoring the progress of these diseases by quantifying the amount of the FDG uptake [21].

6.3.5 Sarcoidosis

Sarcoidosis is the multisystem noncaseating granulomatous disease of unknown etiology affecting any organ of the body. The commonest involvement will be the mediastinal lymphadenopathy followed by lung parenchymal involvement. Here the basis of the uptake is the activated leukocytes, macrophages, lymphocytes with giant cells, which shows proportional uptake to the amount of the activity in these cells. FDG PET-CT is useful for the evaluation depending on the amount of inflammatory activity, the various organs involved, for monitoring the treatment response. Thus, PET-CT is relevant in the morphology–and functional mapping of active inflammatory sites like angle or multiple sites [22–31] (Fig. 6.9).

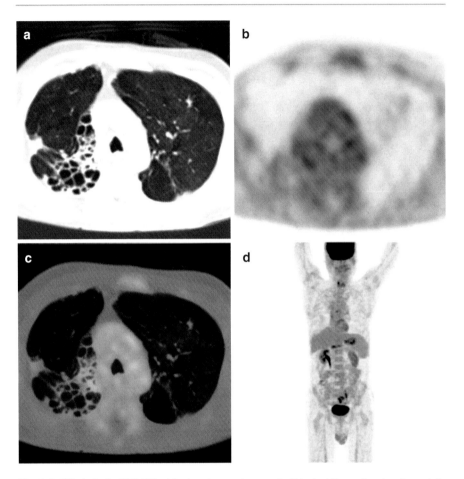

Fig. 6.6 Whole-body PET-CT with chronic cough on and off in last 3 months showing ectatic changes with focal pleural thickening in right upper lobe (**a**) with mild uptake with SUV max of 2 (**b–d**). Rest of the whole body is normal

6.3.5.1 Cystic Fibrosis

Cystic fibrosis is a condition where the neutrophil and macrophage activities are inappropriate and by secreting the pro-inflammatory mediators. This forms the basis of the amount of FDG uptake in this condition. Another aspect of the role of the FDG PET-CT is to identify, quantify, and monitor the airway inflammation [32].

6.3.5.2 Acute Lung Injury and Acute Respiratory Distress Syndrome

Acute lung injury is mostly associated with acute respiratory distress syndrome (ARDS). Here the basis is the neutrophil inflammation due to tissue injury. FDG PET is helpful in giving the information related to the inflammatory response to various stimuli and can demonstrate the pathophysiology of ARI/ARDS [33] (Fig. 6.10).

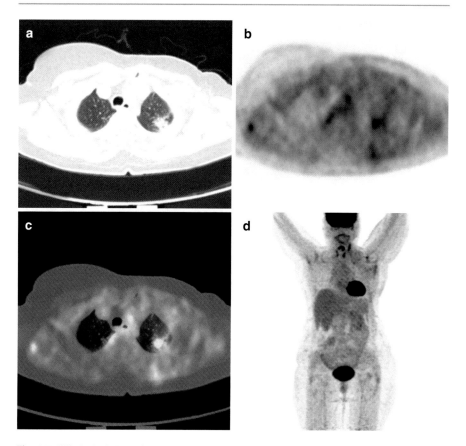

Fig. 6.7 Whole-body PET-CT with fever and weight loss in last 2 months. CT showing small left apical nodular lesion with focal pleural thickening (**a**) consistent with Pulmonary Koch's. PET (**b, d**) and fused images (**c**) show mild tracer activity with SUV max of 3.2 noted

6.3.6   Pulmonary Langerhans Cell Histiocytosis

Langerhans Cell Histiocytosis (LCH) is a rare disease. The etiology is presumed to be abnormal T cell, macrophage, and/or cytokine-mediated process. In this condition, there is releasing of the vascular endothelial growth factor in LCH that leads to the inflammatory changes. Thus, FDG PET-CT is helpful for the evaluation of the LCH for clinical assessment and for monitoring the response to therapy [34].

6.4   Pleural Lesions

This same concept applies to pleural-based lesions. Pleural-based lesions are mostly focal pleural thickening or pleural nodules, pleural mass lesions. The commonest causes of this pleural lesions are tuberculosis, infective

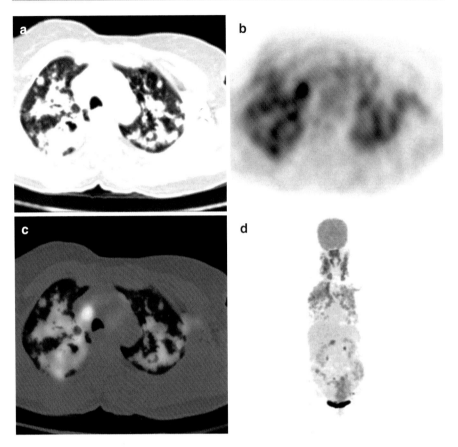

Fig. 6.8 Whole-body PET-CT, CT showing diffuse conglomerate nodular lesions in both lungs with small air bronchogram (**a**) and PET (**b**, **d**) and fused images (**c**) showing mild metabolic activity with SUV max of 6.4. Histopathologically turned out to be Sarcoidosis

inflammatory, collagen diseases, or benign and malignant primary pleural-based lesions. The sensitivity of the pleural-based lesions is again based on SUV max values [35]. The concept is to distinguish between benign and malignant lesions is dual point imaging which distinguishes malignant vs. nonmalignant lesions. FDG PET is equally important in the evaluation of pleural effusions, especially when there is no obvious malignant focus or infective inflammatory focus. Hereby FDG PET-CT subtle focal pleural nodularities can be quantified by SUV max values (Figs. 6.11, 6.12, and 6.13).

The various pathologies in the chest are confined to mediastinum, chest wall, or any concurrent lesions involving chest from the neck or abdomen.

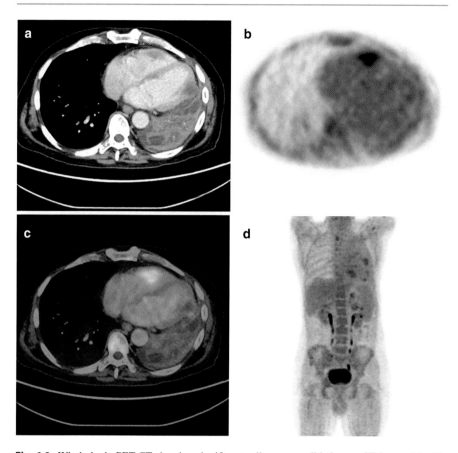

Fig. 6.9 Whole-body PET-CT showing significant collapse consolidation on CT image (**a**) with no metabolic activity on PET images (**b**) and (**d**) and fused image (**c**)

6.5   Mediastinal Lesions

The mediastinal component is either in the form of mediastinal lesions which can be primary mass lesions arising from the mediastinal structures and involving the adjacent structures or vice versa adjacent lesions infiltrating the mediastinum. The other important mediastinal entity is mediastinal nodes. Here mostly the nodes are confined to the drainage areas from the chest. Here the lesions again can be the mediastinal lesions can be primary malignant lesions, secondary malignant lesions in the form of lymphadenopathy. Benign lesions which can be benign neoplasms, collagen diseases, granulomatous diseases, and tuberculosis, and various infective inflammatory pathologies. FDG PET-CT has very important role for evaluation of these lesions and characterizing them depending on the metabolic activity and SUV max values. And the classical presentations of the PET depend on classical features of malignant etiology like mediastinal uptake, necrotic areas, and calcifications. The

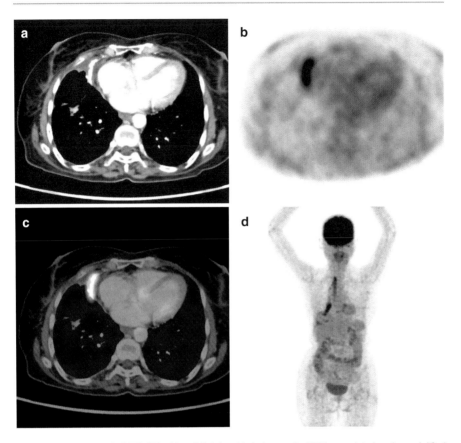

Fig. 6.10 Whole-body PET-CT with mild right-sided chest pain CT image (**a**) showing calcified mediastinal pleural thickening with significant FDG uptake on PET images (**b**) and (**d**) and fused PET-CT image (**c**) with SUV max of 8.6 suggestive of focal chronic calcified pleuritis

same applies here with dual point imaging to differentiate between malignant and nonmalignant pathologies. Most of the oncological work up shows concurrent malignant as well as nonmalignant mediastinal nodes. Here PET-CT plays important role in the evaluation of these structures [36, 37] (Fig. 6.14).

6.6   Chest Wall Lesions

Chest wall lesions comprise again of multiple pathologies like malignant, infective inflammatory, tuberculosis, granulomatous, and significant pathological entities involving skin and subcutaneous planes, muscles, and bones. Separate evaluation of breast parenchyma in females and also in males. The commonest infective inflammatory pathology involving the breast parenchyma is mastitis, gynecomastia in

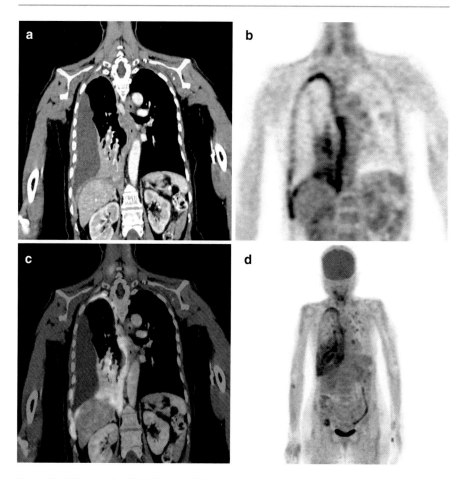

Fig. 6.11 Whole-body PET-CT done CT image (**a**) showing diffuse irregular right costal and mediastinal pleural thickening with moderate pleural effusion and collapse consolidation right lower lobe. PET images (**b**) and (**d**) and fused images (**c**) showing significant uptake with SUV max of 7.7 along the mediastinal pleura in the right lower lobe

males, and to differentiate between benign and malignant nodular lesions involving breast parenchyma (Fig. 6.15). The important infective inflammatory entity involving the chest wall is subcutaneous edema, cellulitis, and focal collection or abscesses in a particular region. FDG PET-CT has an important role in differentiating and evaluating pathologies in the chest wall and sensitive [38–42]. New radiotracers octreotide imaging with or without SPECT CT scan can be useful for the evaluation and monitoring response to therapy (Fig. 6.16).

In the advent PET-MR, the resolution of the chest wall and mediastinal lesions is more defined. One of the biggest advantages of PET-MR is usefulness in the pediatric age group, which we will be discussing in a separate chapter.

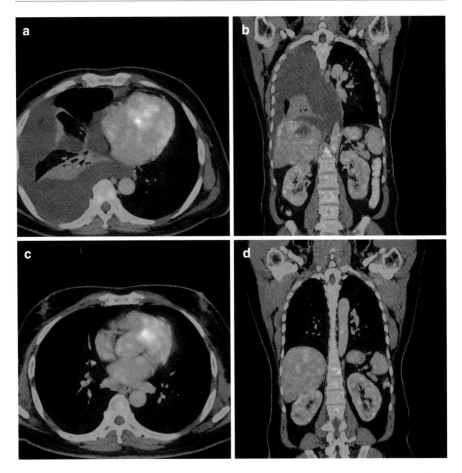

Fig. 6.12 Whole-body PET-CT all (**a**), (**b**), (**c**), and (**d**) fused images of chest showing moderate right pleural effusion with collapse of the lung and no metabolic activity suggestive of nonmalignant pleural effusion

FDG PET is also important for the evaluation of different kinds of pneumoconiosis like silicosis, asbestosis, fibrosis, and other occupational diseases. The basic principle of FDG uptake here is radiotracer deposition in a particular location due to fibroblasts and inflammatory cells [43, 44]. Again, any associated infective inflammatory lung changes can also be diagnosed as a concurrent lesion or as complications due to occupational diseases.

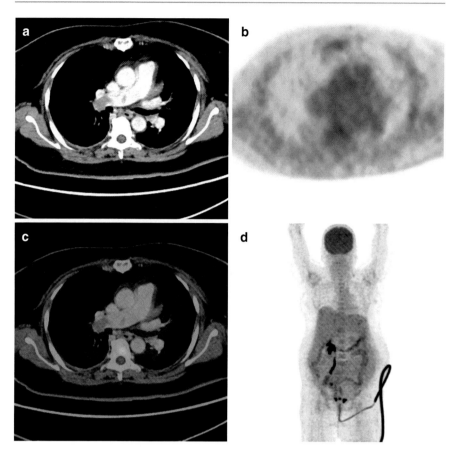

Fig. 6.13 Whole-body PET-CT with chest sections CT image showing intraluminal thrombus in main right pulmonary artery (**a**) with no FDG uptake on PET images (**b**) and (**d**) and fused images (**c**) suggestive of chronic nonreactive pulmonary thromboembolism

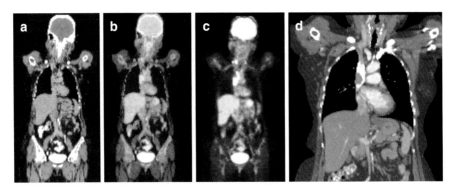

Fig. 6.14 Whole-body PET-CT showing intraluminal thrombus in superior vena cava in Contrast CT image (**a**, **d**), which is corresponding with the uptake on FDG in PET image (**c**) and fused image (**b**). Image (**a**) Non-contrast CT image does not show any specific thrombus

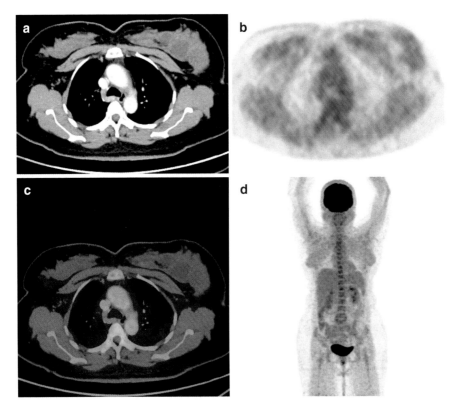

Fig. 6.15 Whole-body PET-CT of 43-year-old female CT image (**a**) showing lobulated cystic lesions in the left breast. PET images (**b**) and (**d**) and fused image (**c**) showing FDG uptake. Features suggestive of fibrocystic disease left breast

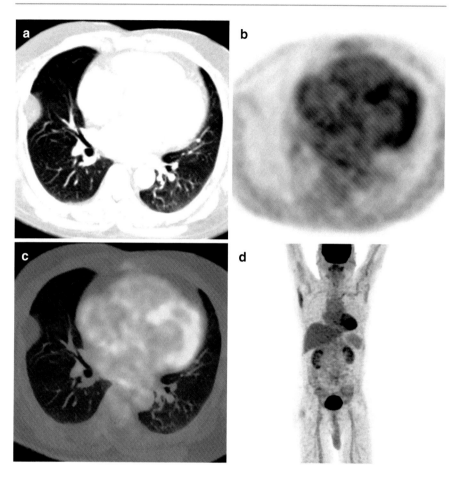

Fig. 6.16 Whole-body PET-CT CT image (**a**) showing focal nodular pleural-based lesion with the erosion of rib along the right costal pleura with no FDG uptake on PET image (**b**) and (**d**) and fused image (**c**) suggestive of chronic infective inflammatory nodule

References

1. Basu S, Hess S, Braad P-EN, et al. The basic principles of FDG-PET/CT imaging. PET Clin. 2014;9(4):355–70, v.
2. Akdis M, Burgler S, Crameri R, Eiwegger T, Fujita H, Gomez E, et al. Interleukins, from 1 to 37, and interferon-gamma: receptors, functions, and roles in diseases. J Allergy Clin Immunol. 2011;127(e1–70):701–21.
3. Scheller J, Garbers C, Rose-John S. Interleukin-6: from basic biology to selective blockade of pro-inflammatory activities. Semin Immunol. 2014;26:2–12.
4. Petho G, Reeh PW. Sensory and signaling mechanisms of bradykinin, eicosanoids, platelet-activating factor, and nitric oxide in peripheral nociceptors. Physiol Rev. 2012;92:1699–775.
5. Cochran BJ, Ryder WJ, Parmar A, et al. Determining glucose metabolism kinetics using 18F-FDG micro-PET/CT. J Vis Exp. 2017;(123):55184.
6. Jones HA, Cadwallader KA, White JF, et al. Dissociation between respiratory burst activity and deoxyglucose uptake in human neutrophil granulocytes: implications for interpretation of 18F-FDG PET images. J Nucl Med. 2002;43:652–7.
7. Kubota R, Yamada S, Kubota K, Ishiwata K, Tamahashi N, Ido T. Intratumoral distribution of fluorine-18-fluorodeoxyglucose in-vivo: high accumulation in macrophages and granulation tissues studied by micro-autoradiography. J Nucl Med. 1992;33:1972–80.
8. Dimastromatteo J, Charles EJ, Laubach LE. Molecular imaging of pulmonary diseases. Respir Res. 2018;19:1–17.
9. Kim IJ, Lee JS, Kim SJ, et al. Double-phase 18F-FDG PET-CT for determination of pulmonary tuberculoma activity. Eur J Nucl Med Mol Imaging. 2008;35:808–14.
10. Abe M, Kobashi Y, Mouri K, et al. Solitary pulmonary nodule due to Mycobacterium kansasii. Intern Med. 2011;50:775–8.
11. Soussan M, Brillet PY, Mekinian A, et al. Patterns of pulmonary tuberculosis on FDG-PET/CT. Eur J Radiol. 2012;81:2872–6.
12. Demura Y, Tsuchida T, Uesaka D, et al. Usefulness of 18F-fluorodeoxyglucose positron emission tomography for diagnosing disease activity and monitoring therapeutic response in patients with pulmonary mycobacteriosis. Eur J Nucl Med Mol Imaging. 2009;36:632–9.
13. Sathekge MM, Maes A, Pottel H, Stoltz A, van de Wiele C. Dual time-point FDG PET-CT for differentiating benign from malignant solitary pulmonary nodules in a TB endemicarea. S Afr Med J. 2010;100:598–601.
14. Shin L, Katz DS, Yung E. Hypermetabolism on F-18 FDG PET of multiple pulmonary nodules resulting from bronchiolitis obliterans organizing pneumonia. Clin Nucl Med. 2004;29:654–6.
15. Gambhir S, Ravina M, Rangan K, Dixit M, Barai S, Bomanji J. International atomic energy agency extra-pulmonary TB consortium. Imaging in extrapulmonary tuberculosis. Int J Infect Dis. 2017;56:237–47.
16. Chiu C-F, Liu Y-Y, Hsu W-H, et al. Shorter-time dual-phase FDG PET/CT in characterizing solid or ground-glass nodules based on surgical results. Clin Imaging. 2012;36:509–14. https://doi.org/10.1016/j.clinimag.2011.11.032.
17. Lee HY, Lee KS, Han J, Kim BT, Cho YS, Shim YM, et al. Mucinous versus non-mucinous solitary pulmonary nodular bronchioloalveolar carcinoma: CT and FDG PET findings and pathologic comparisons. Lung Cancer. 2009;65:170–5.
18. Nakajo M, Jinguji M, Aoki M, et al. The clinical value of texture analysis of dual-time-point 18F-FDG-PET/CT imaging to differentiate between 18F-FDG-avid benign and malignant pulmonary lesions. Eur Radiol. 2020;30(3):1759–69.
19. Sheikhbahaei S, Mena E, Marcus C, et al. 18F-FDG PET/CT: therapy response assessment interpretation (Hopkins criteria) and survival outcomes in lung cancer patients. J Nucl Med. 2016;57:855–60.
20. Jones HA, Marino PS, Shakur BH, et al. In vivo assessment of lung inflammatory cell activity in patients with COPD and asthma. Eur Respir J. 2003;21:567–73.
21. Kothekar E, Borja AJ, Gerke O, Werner TJ, Alavi A, Revheim ME. Assessing respiratory muscle activity with 18F-FDG-PET/CT in patients with COPD. Am J Nucl Med Mol Imaging. 2019;9:309–15.

22. Reichert M, Bensadoun ES. PET imaging in patients with coal workers pneumoconiosis and suspected malignancy. J Thorac Oncol. 2009;4:649–51.

23. Nishiyama Y, Yamamoto Y, Fukunaga K, Takinami H, Iwado Y, Satoh K, Ohkawa M. Comparative evaluation of 18F-FDG PET and 67Ga scintigraphy in patients with sarcoidosis. J Nucl Med. 2006;47:1571–6.

24. Norikane T, Yamamoto Y, Maeda Y, Noma T, Dobashi H, Nishiyama Y. Comparative evaluation of 18F-FLT and 18F-FDG for detecting cardiac and extra-cardiac thoracic involvement in patients with newly diagnosed sarcoidosis. EJNMMI Res. 2017;7:69.

25. Palestro CJ, Schultz BL, Horowitz M, Swyer AJ. Indium-111-leukocyte and gallium-67 imaging in acute sarcoidosis: report of two patients. J Nucl Med. 1992;33:2027–9.

26. Rizzato G, Blasi A. A European survey on the usefulness of 67Ga lung scans in assessing sarcoidosis. Experience in 14 research centers in seven different countries. Ann N Y Acad Sci. 1986;465:463–78.

27. Israel HL, Albertine KH, Park CH. Whole-body gallium 67 scans. Role in diagnosis of sarcoidosis. Am Rev Respir Dis. 1991;144:1182–6.

28. Sulavik SB, Spencer RP, Weed DA, Shapiro HR, Shiue HR, Castriotta RJ. Recognition of distinctive patterns of gallium-67 distribution in sarcoidosis. J Nucl Med. 1990;31:1909–14.

29. Sulavik SB, Spencer RP, Palestro CJ, Swyer AJ, Teirstein AS, Goldsmith SJ. Specificity and sensitivity of distinctive chest radiographic and/or 67 Ga images in the non-invasive diagnosis of sarcoidosis. Chest. 1993;103:403–9.

30. Braun JJ, Kessler R, Constantinesco A, et al. 18F-FDG PET/CT in sarcoidosis management: review and report of 20 cases. Eur J Nucl Med Mol Imaging. 2008;35:1537–43.

31. Kiatboonsri C, Resnick SC, Chan KM, et al. The detection of recurrent sarcoidosis by FDG-PET in a lung transplant recipient. West J Med. 1998;168:130–2.

32. Keijsers RG, Verzijlbergen FJ, Oyen WJ, et al. 18F-FDG PET, genotype-corrected ACE and sIL-2R in newly diagnosed sarcoidosis. Eur J Nucl Med Mol Imaging. 2009;36:1131–7.

33. Konstan MW, Berger M. Current understanding of the inflammatory process in cystic fibrosis: onset and etiology. Pediatr Pulmonol. 1997;24:137–42.

34. Braune J, Hofheinz F, Bluth T, Kiss T, Wittenstein J, Scharffenberg M, Kotzerke J, Gamade Abreu M. Comparison of static 18F-FDG-PET/CT (SUV, SUR) and dynamic 18F-FDGPET/CT(Ki) for quantification of pulmonary inflammation in acute lung injury. J Nucl Med. 2019;60:1629–34.

35. Kannourakis G, Abbas A. The role of cytokines in the pathogenesis of Langerhans cell histiocytosis. Br J Cancer Suppl. 1994;23:S37–40.

36. Kaira K, Serizawa M, Koh Y, Takahashi T, Hanaoka H, Oriuchi N, et al. Relationship between 18F-FDG uptake on positron emission tomography and molecular biology in malignant pleural mesothelioma. Eur J Cancer. 2012;48:1244–54.

37. Hara T, Inagaki K, Kosaka N, Morita T. Sensitive detection of mediastinal lymphnode metastasis of lung cancer with 11C-choline PET. J Nucl Med. 2000;41:1507–13.

38. Tatci E, Ozmen O, Dadali Y, et al. The role of FDG PET/CT in evaluation of mediastinal masses and neurogenic tumors of chest wall. Int J Clin Exp Med. 2015;8(7):11146–52.

39. Moore SL, Rafii M. Imaging of musculoskeletal and spinal tuberculosis. Radiol Clin North Am. 2001;39:329–42.

40. Yago Y, Yukihiro M, Kuroki H, et al. Cold tuberculous abscess identified by FDG PET. Ann Nucl Med. 2005;19:515–51.

41. Harkirat S, Anana SS, Indrajit LK, Dash AK. Pictorial essay: PET/CT in tuberculosis. Indian J Radiol Imaging. 2008;18:141–7.

42. Litmanovich D, Gourevich K, Israel O, Gallimidi Z. Unexpected foci of 18F-FDG uptake in the breast detected by PET/CT: incidence and clinical significance. Eur J Nucl Med Mol Imaging. 2009;36(10):1558–64.

43. O'Connell M, Kennedy M. Progressive massive fibrosis secondary to pulmonary silicosis appearance on F-18 fluorodeoxyglucose PET/CT. Clin Nucl Med. 2004;29(11):754–5.

44. Choi EK, Park HL, Yoo IR. The clinical value of F-18 FDG PET/CT in differentiating malignant from benign lesions in pneumoconiosis patients. Eur Radiol. 2020;30(1):442–51.

PET-CT in Myocardium, Epicardium, and Pericardium Infective Inflammatory Pathologies

7

Key Points

FDG PET-CT is important in the evaluation and diagnosis of the various infections involving pericardium, myocardium, and endocardium.

With the advent of PET-CT technology, it is helpful in the evaluation of prosthetic heart valves, stents, grafts, and cardiac implantable electronic devices.

With a lot of studies, PET-CT plays important role in the acquisition, semi-quantification, and interpretation of various pathologies.

7.1   Introduction

Infective inflammatory conditions of the heart are important subject of conditions that comes under the PUO/FUO. Predominant infective pathologies are pericarditis, myocarditis, and endocarditis. Pericardium very thin structure too difficult to evaluate exact pathology by conventional imaging modalities like CT and MR. But with technological advantages, CT and MR impacts good imaging modalities but the only difference with the PET is the functional imaging component. Prosthetic materials and valves replacements, grafts, implantable devices like pacemakers and other predisposing factors involving endocarditis needs to be meticulously evalauted. The excellent role of FDG PET-CT in infections of the heart has been reviewed in detail by Miller and colleagues [1, 2]. Patient preparation and imaging the heart is challenging because of continuous movement or mobility of the heart, for this some preparation has to be done to evaluate the heart. Many protocols have been set but not one has been set as a standard protocol. However, recent recommendations by the Japanese Society of Nuclear Cardiology agreed that a low carbohydrate fat diet and prolong fasting can be considered but still it is debatable [3–6]. The main problem here is to suppress the myocardial glucose metabolism which may give many false positive results which are common and this needs to be nullified as far as possible (Fig. 7.1).

S. Shaikh, *PET-CT in Infection and Inflammation*,
https://doi.org/10.1007/978-981-15-9801-2_7

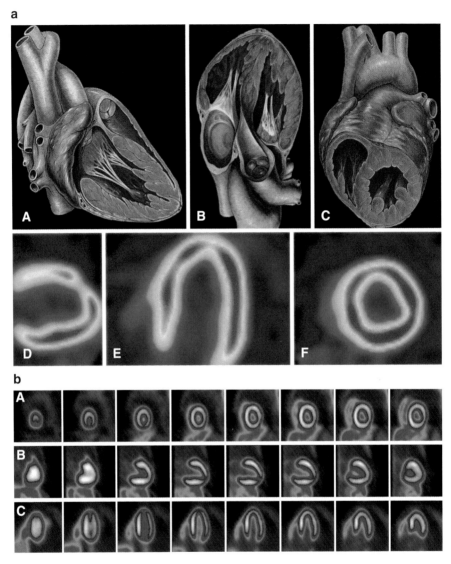

Fig. 7.1 (**a**): (A) Corresponding to PET (D). (B) Corresponding to PET (E). (C) Corresponding to PET (F). Normal sections of PET myocardium. (**b**): Normal ammonia cardiac scan images in horizontal, short and long axis

7.2   Pericarditis

Pericarditis is the inflammation of the pericardium, which has varied range of clinical presentations like chest pain, palpitations, shortness of breath, and symptoms mimicking myocardial infarction or ischemia. The other symptoms may include fever, weight loss, and fatigue. With this significant overlap of symptoms, it is difficult to distinguish between myocarditis, pericarditis, and vasculitis. CT and MRI already have a significant role in the analysis and assessment of structural abnormalities of this cardiovascular system. PET-CT plays an important role in the evaluation of pericardial and myocardial pathology. FDG PET has a unique ability to identify the metabolic activity of the pericardium and myocardium. Now, FDG PET has become a valuable tool to evaluate in patients who present with systemic symptoms [7–10]. The biggest drawback of FDG PET-CT is the radiotracer accumulation in the normal myocardium. This is again more prominently seen in the left ventricular myocardium because of greater muscle mass. The sequence of uptake in cardiac chamber is left ventricle, right ventricle, right atrium, and left atrium. This physiologic uptake in normal myocardium varies from diffuse or focal uptake in the same person depending on various physiological conditions, fasting state, and other parameters. Pericardial uptake is not seen unless and until there is inflammation, thickening, or pathology of pericardium, which can be focal or diffuse. The preparation criteria are a low carbohydrate diet with 12 h minimum fasting to suppress the normal physiological uptake in normal myocytes. Pericarditis can be diffuse pericardial thickening, focal pericardial thickening, pericardial tumor, pericardial calcification and combination of these findings and the most important cause is tuberculosis. The amount of uptake in the pericardium is directly proportional to the amount of active inflammation. Thus, FDG PET-CT can differentiate between acute and chronic pericarditis [11, 12]. The real issue comes with pericardial nodule vs. pericardial tumor. Here, the dual time point imaging may help to a certain extent. The commonest pathology tuberculosis mimics most of the time with the malignant pathology. Constrictive pericarditis usually not having significant uptake but is crucial to diagnose for it may complicate pericardial tamponade (Figs. 7.2, 7.3, and 7.4).

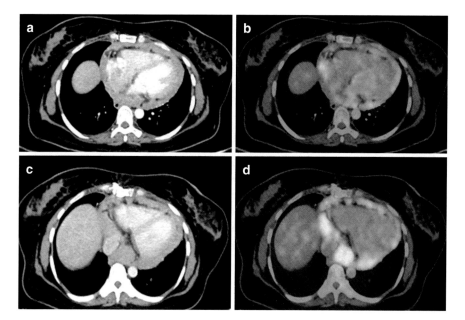

Fig. 7.2 Whole-body PET-CT at the level of cardia CT image (**a**) and (**c**) showing irregular nodular pericardial thickening with associated mild effusion and PET-CT fused (**b**) and (**d**) with SUV max of 7.2. Findings are suggestive of constrictive pericarditis

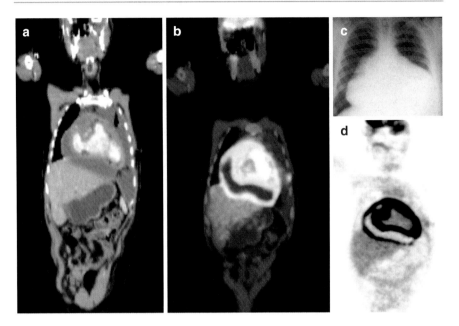

Fig. 7.3 Whole-body CT image (**a**) showing pericardial thickening with moderate pericardial effusion. Image (**b**) and (**d**) showing diffuse pericardial uptake with no uptake in the inferior aspect due to fluid accumulation by gravity. Image (**c**) Chest radiograph showing flask shape heart. Features suggestive of pericardial effusion

7.3   Myocarditis

Myocardial diseases causing myocarditis most commonly are inflammatory cardiomyopathies, sarcoidosis, eosinophilic disease, and other infective causes of myocarditis. FDG PET is important to evaluate the direct assessment of infiltrative processes of the myocardium. FDG PET identifies the focal or diffuse area of metabolic activity or inactivity. The protocol for PET myocardial imaging can be rest or stress or can be both. The role of FDG PET is for initial diagnosis and monitoring response to treatment. The basic pathophysiology of myocarditis is an injury to cardiac myocytes causing inflammation, cell necrosis, degeneration, or a combination of these three. As described the commonest cause of myocarditis are viral infections, autoimmune process, cardiotoxic agents, and hypersensitivity reactions. Post radiation and post chemotherapy may also show diffuse metabolic activity consistent with myocarditis (Fig. 7.5).

7.4   Epi-Pericarditis

This condition mimics acute pleuritic chest pain. Clinically nonspecific symptoms of myocardial infarction of pericarditis. It can be focal or diffuse and associated with epi-pericardial fat necrosis. This mimics on FDG PET-CT as an inflammatory process. The other associated conditions are epi-pericardial fat necrosis. FDG

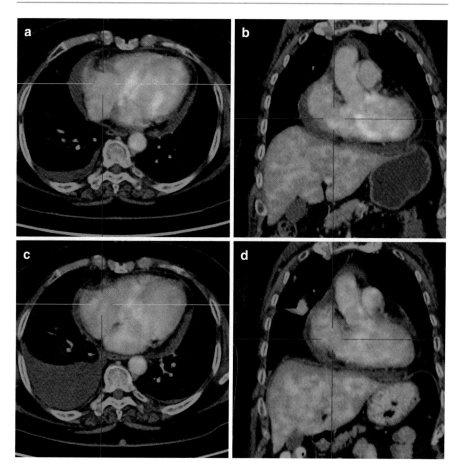

Fig. 7.4 Whole-body PET-CT images (**a**), (**b**), (**c**), and (**d**) at the level of cardia showing mild pericardial thickening and pericardial effusion. No FDG uptake. Moderate right pleural effusion noted with no FDG uptake

PET-CT at this level shows fat-containing mass. Small conditions like lipomatous hypertrophy of the interatrial septum may also mimick this condition. In this condition, FDG PET-CT shows focal area of increased metabolic activity in the interatrial septum. Atherosclerosis is also an important entity associated with chronic inflammatory changes to the intimal layer of vascular endothelium. This atherosclerosis affects all the vessels with varying degrees of involvement depending on the atherosclerotic plaque, wall thickening, luminal stenosis, or enlargement. FDG PET-CT may show no uptake, mild diffuse uptake, or focal increased uptake along the walls. FDG PET plays important role in the evaluation of coronary arteries and their branches which shows a significant amount of atherosclerosis from soft plaque that is non-obstructing to highly calcified near complete or complete stenosis of the walls [13–15]. This involvement of the coronary arteries is the direct reflection of the myocardial involvement. FDG PET-CT along with the other imaging parameters like CT coronary angiogram and CT aortogram shows complementary analysis.

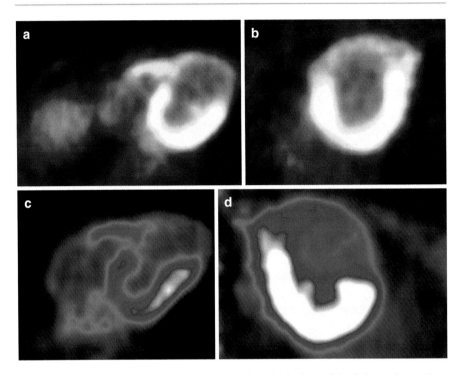

Fig. 7.5 FDG PET scan showing LAD stenosis territory in the form of the defect in the uptake

7.5   Ammonia Imaging

Ammonia is the most precise radiotracer with a short half-life of 2.2 min. This radiotracer has to be injected immediately after the production if the cyclotron is onsite because of very short half-life of ammonia. This radiotracer is more specific and precise for cardiac imaging and more sensitive in diagnostic accuracy compared with routine FDG scan. Along with ammonia N-13, rubidium 82 is also an equally sensitive radiotracer for the evaluation of myocardial perfusion. With this two-radiotracer myocardial perfusion stress is performed which is more sensitive compared to the FDG PET scan (Figs. 7.6, 7.7, 7.8, and 7.9).

Other radiotracers used are 62 Cu—PTSM, 62-zink 15O, 18F—Flurpiridaz of varying half-life are being used.

7.6   Artifacts in Cardiac PET-CT

PET-CT has some artifacts in relation to misalignment between CT and PET data caused by patient movement, cardiac motion, or respiratory motion. This can lead to defects in the evaluation giving false-positive results. Another technical artifact is because of scintillating crystals. Detection of multivessel coronary artery disease can be identified by CT or DSA angiogram. This CT or DSA angiogram finding has to be correlated to measure the myocardial blood flow reflecting the myocardial perfusion quantification. Sometimes, hybrid PET with coronary CT angiogram at one go can be done for better evalaution and simultaneous correlation.

7.7   Native Valve Endocarditis

FDG PET-CT is not much value with reduced sensitivity in the valve endocarditis. In a recent study of 115 patients with suspected valve endocarditis reported a sensitivity of 22% [10, 16]. Though the specificity is high, the diagnostic accuracy is low. The reason for this is due to small vegetations on valve leaflets. These vegetations are small and more important. The reason is WBC response to bacteria. The basic principle of FDG PET-CT depends on white cell migration and glucose consumption, which is directly proportional to the disease. Positive FDG PET-CT findings may indicate more complicated infection with the involvement of adjacent valve structures. However, new PET-CT studies related to infectious foci show the probability of 55% of patient involvement [17]. However, with the advent high-resolution PET-CT more and more studies are coming up for these valvular pathologies.

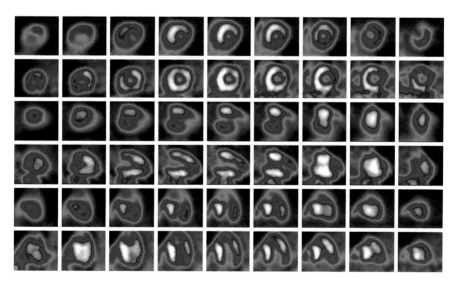

Fig. 7.6 Ammonia scan with images in all three axis showing ischemia in apical and mid-anterior apical lateral wall myocardial infection in apical inferior wall

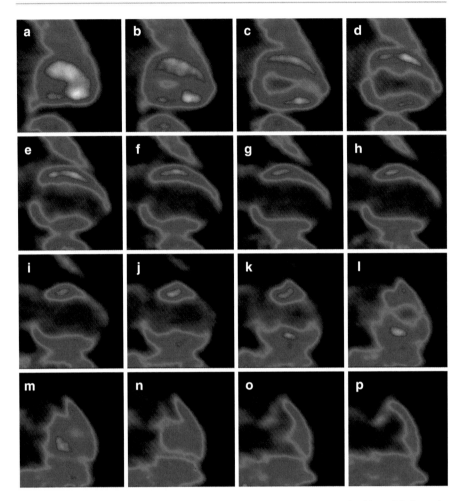

Fig. 7.7 Reduced perfusion in the apex and apical inferior wall with no significant FDG uptake on PET scan. No viable myocardium

7.8   Cardiac Implantable Devices

7.8.1   Imaging

Cardiac implantable electronic devices are seen with varying amounts of infection. This is because of coexisting infection which is difficult to diagnose by routine investigative modalities. A recent meta-analysis study from 2019 reported a sensitivity of 83% and specificity of 89% [18–22]. With this FDG PET-CT has a sensitivity of 96% and specificity of 97%. The associated physiological myocardial uptake has to be interpreted along the cardiac portion of the leads. The infection can be in the form of vegetations and may not have much leukocyte response. A recent study

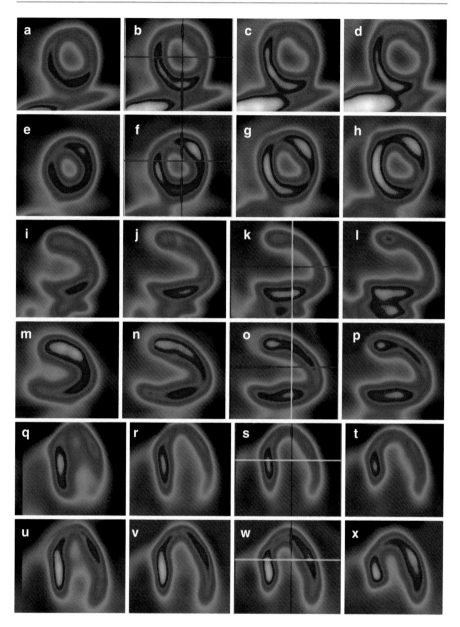

Fig. 7.8 Reduced perfusion in apical anterior and basal lateral wall, which shows FDG uptake in PET scan. Viable myocardium

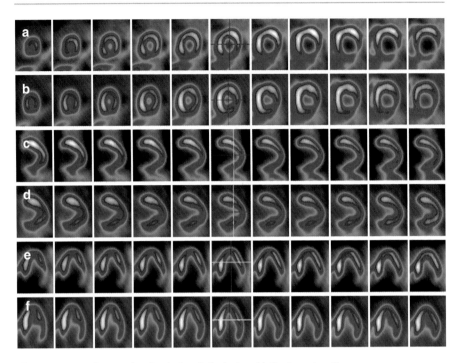

Fig. 7.9 Ammonia scan showing ischemia in the basal inferolateral wall

with clinical suspicion of implantable device infection showed FDG PET-CT reclassified nearly 1 in 4 patients when added to duke criteria. With this, it was able to diagnose endocarditis in suspected cases of infection and also in the possible cases of rejection.

7.8.2   Left Ventricular Device Infection

The left ventricular devices are the form of implantable devices that perform the circulatory function of the heart. They typically consist of a percutaneous pump that is connected to the circulation via an inflow cannula. A recent case series and meta-analysis of FDG PET-CT in LVAD infections published in July 2019 showed a significant amount of sensitivity of 92% and specificity of 83% for the detection of LVAD infection [23–25]. The sensitivity of FDG PET-CT was higher compared to leukocyte labeled scintigraphy. The sensitivity of PET-CT was significantly higher 95 vs. 71%. The reason for false-positive results is due to surgical adhesions to reinforce the inflow and outflow cannulas. Dense structure pump housing is equally prone to beam hardening and scattering of low-dose CT. The value of multimodality imaging with the advent of FDG PET-CT to identify infection is important. As explained, the vegetation cannot be effectively ruled out with FDG PET-CT alone. So, other imaging modalities like 2D echo, trans-thoracic echocardiography, and trans-esophageal echocardiography cannot distinguish the infective foci on the devices or prosthetic valves. CT Angiogram also having increasing sensitivity and specificity of 86.4 and 87.5% for FDG PET-CT with significantly increases to 91 and 90.6% for combined FDG PET and CT angiogram [26–28]. With this, all imaging modalities have their own advantages and disadvantages for the evaluation of device infection. This multimodality imaging is especially valuable and should be evaluated in multidisciplinary settings. The imaging acquisition protocols whole-body imaging protocol should be the most preferred protocol to rule out infective foci in the extremity. The evaluation of intracranial lesions is difficult due to the physiological uptake of FDG in the background myocardial activity. Additional gated images of the cardiac region are of additional value for visualization of cardiac and valve motion through the cardiac cycle and faster, easy, and better compared with CT angiogram images. The current European Society of Cardiology guidelines specify the use of FDG PET-CT in the first 3 months of surgery to be discouraged due to false-positive results. This false-positive result is due to inflammation during the healing process [29–32].

7.9 Interpretation

In general, the strongest predictor of infection is the focal uptake of FDG, which is not physiologically noted. The common area of uptake involves the valve leaflets, valve annuli, or prosthetic material. The issue of mechanical prosthetic valves and bioprosthetic valves, the amount of uptake is not the same and has to be differentiated with the normal variants of uptake, especially in the cases where the uptake is mild in intensity. In caveat, the significant high uptake in prosthetic valves or with clinical suspicion of infections, this focus can be interpreted as a possible infection. In cases with vascular grafts, surgical postoperative adhesions are more common in other implants and should be high uptake even along the edges of the implants or close to insertion into the graph. Reverse is no uptake in FDG does mean no evidence of disease or no vegetations. However, FDG avid infective foci like septic lung emboli for right-sided disease and mycotic aneurysms can be more convenient feature of endocarditis. Artifacts may arise due to high-density beam hardening or scatter artifacts on the low dose CT. Other intracardiac pathologies like cardiac tumors or intraluminal thrombus to be also evaluated (Fig. 7.10).

7.10 Future Perspective

The most important problem with FDG PET-CT is to develop a uniform guideline regarding the standardized reading, interpretation, measurement, and report of these findings. The newer use of semi-quantification is not specific due to various criteria mentioned by different centers or associations. Again, the guidelines may vary with different prostheses and different types of devices like valves, stents, and prosthetic materials.

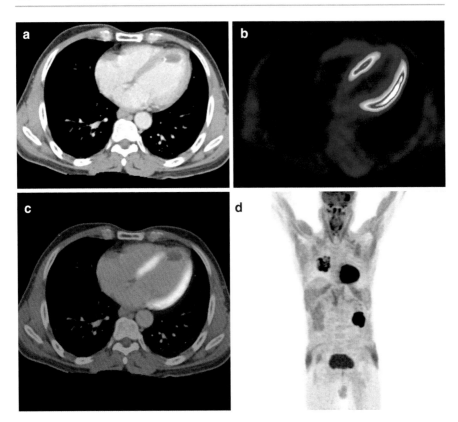

Fig. 7.10 Whole-body PET-CT done for carcinoma right lung showing intraluminal thrombus in the left ventricle with no FDG uptake suggestive of chronic inactive thrombus

7.11   Conclusion

With the integrated PET-CT for cardiac imaging, it has become easier to detect and quantify the plaque vascular reactivity, endothelial status, coronary artery evaluation, evaluation of epicardium, pericardium, myocardium, and endocardium for various radiotracers. The futuristic PET-CT will be targeted molecular imaging for diagnosis and therapeutic.

References

1. Millar BC, de Camargo RA, Alavi A, et al. PET/computed tomography evaluation of infection of the heart. PET Clin. 2019;14(2):251–69.
2. Millar BC, Prendergast BD, Alavi A, et al. [18]FDG- positron emission tomography (PET) has a role to play in the diagnosis and therapy of infective endocarditis and cardiac device infection. Int J Cardiol. 2013;167:1724–36.

3. Habib G, Lancellotti P, Antunes MJ, et al. 2015 ESC guidelines for the management of infective endocarditis: the task force for the management of infective endocarditis of the European Society of Cardiology (ESC). endorsed by: European Association for Cardio-Thoracic Surgery (EACTS), the European Association of Nuclear Medicine (EANM). Eur Heart J. 2015;36:3075–128.

4. Millar BC, Habib G, Moore JE. New diagnostic approaches in infective endocarditis. Heart. 2016;102:796–807.

5. Balmforth D, Chacko J, Uppal R. Does positron emission tomography/computed tomography aid the diagnosis of prosthetic valve infective endocarditis? Interact Cardiovasc Thorac Surg. 2016;23:648–52.

6. Camargo RA, Siciliano RF, Paixao MR, et al. Diagnostic value of positron emission tomography (PET/ CT) in native and prosthetic infective endocarditis. Eur Heart J. 2017;38(Issue Suppl 1):1010.

7. Adler Y, Charron P, Imazio M, et al. 2015 ESC guidelines for the diagnosis and management of pericardial diseases: the task force for the diagnosis and management of pericardial diseases of the European Society of Cardiology (ESC) endorsed by: the European Association for Cardio-Thoracic Surgery (EACTS). Eur Heart J. 2015;36:2921–64.

8. Assayag M, Abbas R, Chanson N, et al. Diagnosis of systemic inflammatory diseases among patients admitted for acute pericarditis with pericardial effusion. J Cardiovasc Med (Hagerstown). 2017;18:875–80.

9. Lobert P, Brown RK, Dvorak RA, Corbett JR, Kazerooni EA, Wong KK. Spectrum of physiological and pathological cardiac and pericardial uptake of FDG in oncology PET-CT. Clin Radiol. 2013;68:e59–71.

10. Dong A, Dong H, Wang Y, Cheng C, Zuo C, Lu J. (18) F-FDG PET/CT in differentiating acute tuberculous from idiopathic pericarditis: preliminary study. Clin Nucl Med. 2013;38(4):e160–5.

11. Sagristà-Sauleda J, Mercé J, Permanyer-Miralda G, Soler-Soler J. Clinical clues to the causes of large pericardial effusions. Am J Med. 2000;109(2):95–101.

12. Vaidyanathan S, Patel CN, Scarsbrook AF, Chowdhury FU. FDG PET/CT in infection and inflammation—current and emerging clinical applications. Clin Radiol. 2015;70(7):787–800.

13. Imazio M, Cecchi E, Demichelis B, Ierna S, Demarie D, Ghisio A, et al. Indicators of poor prognosis of acute pericarditis. Circulation. 2007;115(21):2739–44.

14. Fukuchi K, Ohta H, Matsumura K, et al. Benign variations and incidental abnormalities of myocardial FDG uptake in the fasting state as encountered during routine oncology positron emission tomography studies. Br J Radiol. 2007;80(949):3–11.

15. Cheng VY, Slomka PJ, Ahlen M, Thomson LE, Waxman AD, Berman DS. Impact of carbohydrate restriction with and without fatty acid loading on myocardial 18F-FDG uptake during PET: a randomized controlled trial. J Nucl Cardiol. 2010;17(2):286–91.

16. de Camargo RA, Bitencourt MS, Meneghetti JC, et al. The role of 18F-FDG-PET/CT in the diagnosis of left-sided endocarditis: native vs. prosthetic valves endocarditis. Clin Infect Dis. 2019;70(4):583–94.

17. Swart LE, Gomes A, Scholtens AM, et al. Improving the diagnostic performance of ^{18}F-FDG PET/CT in prosthetic heart valve endocarditis. Circulation. 2018;138:1412–27.

18. Kouijzer IJE, Berrevoets MAH, Aarntzen EHJG, et al. 18F-fluorodeoxyglucose positron-emission tomography combined with computed tomography as a diagnostic tool in native valve endocarditis. Nucl Med Commun. 2018;39(8):747–52.

19. Granados U, Fuster D, Pericas JM, et al. Diagnostic accuracy of ^{18}F-FDG PET/CT in infective endocarditis and implantable cardiac electronic device infection: a cross-sectional study. J Nucl Med. 2016;57:1726–32.

20. Mikail N, Benali K, Mahida B, et al. ^{18}F-FDG-PET/ CT imaging to diagnose septic emboli and mycotic aneurysms in patients with endocarditis and cardiac device infections. Curr Cardiol Rep. 2018;20:14.

21. Mahmood M, Kendi AT, Farid S, et al. Role of (18)F- FDG PET/CT in the diagnosis of cardiovascular implantable electronic device infections: a meta- analysis. J Nucl Cardiol. 2019;26(3):958–70.

22. Kusumoto FM, Schoenfeld MH, Wilkoff BL. HRS expert consensus statement on cardio-vascular implantable electronic device lead management and extraction. Heart Rhythm. 2017;14:e503–51.
23. Sarrazin JF, Philippon F, Tessier M, et al. Usefulness of fluorine-18 positron emission tomography/ computed tomography for identification of cardio- vascular implantable electronic device infections. J Am Coll Cardiol. 2012;59:1616–25.
24. Tam MC, Patel VN, Weinberg RL, et al. Diagnostic accuracy of FDG PET/CT in suspected LVAD infections: a case series, systematic review, and meta- analysis. JACC Cardiovasc Imaging. 2019;13(5):1191–202.
25. Legallois D, Manrique A. Diagnosis of infection in patients with left ventricular assist device: PET or SPECT? J Nucl Cardiol. 2018;26(1):56–8. https://doi.org/10.1007/s12350-018-1324-6.
26. Absi M, Bocchini C, Price JF, et al. F-fluorodeoxyglucose positive emission tomography/CT imaging for left ventricular assist device-associated infections in children. Cardiol Young. 2018;28:1157–9.
27. Avramovic N, Dell'Aquila AM, Weckesser M, et al. Metabolic volume performs better than SUVmax inthe detection of left ventricular assist device drive- line infection. Eur J Nucl Med Mol Imaging. 2017;44:1870–7.
28. Bernhardt AM, Pamirsad MA, Brand C, et al. The value of fluorine-18 deoxyglucose positron emission tomography scans in patients with ventricular assist device specific infections. Eur J Cardiothorac Surg. 2017;51:1072–7.
29. Akin S, Muslem R, Constantinescu AA, et al. ^{18}F-FDG PET/CT in the diagnosis and manage-ment of continuous flow left ventricular assist device infections: a case series and review of the literature. ASAIO J. 2018;64:e11–9.
30. Habib G, Lancellotti P, Antunes MJ, et al. ESC guidelines for the management of infective endo-carditis: the task force for the management of infective endocarditis of the European Society of Cardiology (ESC) endorsed by: European Association for Cardio-Thoracic Surgery (EACTS), the European Association of Nuclear Medicine (EANM). Eur Heart J. 2015;36(44):3075–128.
31. Herzog BA, Husmann L, Valenta I, et al. Long-term prognostic value of 13N-ammonia myo-cardial perfusion positron emission tomography added value of coronary flow reserve. J Am Coll Cardiol. 2009;54:150–6. https://doi.org/10.1016/j.jacc.2009.02.069.
32. Sampson UK, Dorbala S, Limaye A, et al. Diagnostic accuracy of rubidium-82 myocardial per-fusion imaging with hybrid positron emission tomography/computed tomography in the detec-tion of coronary artery disease. J Am Coll Cardiol. 2007;49:1052–8. https://doi.org/10.1016/j.jacc.2006.12.015.

PET-CT in Cardiovascular Pathologies

8

Key Points

Cardiovascular disorders are one of the leading causes of death worldwide and are the biggest challenge for modern medicine. Despite a lot of advances, the prevention and management of cardiovascular disorders are the biggest challenge. With the advent of various Molecular Imaging modalities, PET-CT has been well established as an important modality for the evaluation of various conditions. PET-CT can evaluate both anatomical and metabolic changes in a variety of infective inflammatory and myocardial disorders. Myocardial perfusion imaging effectively evaluates the coronary vascularity and other diffuse cardiac involvement. There are a lot of advancements in the diagnosis, treatment, prevention, and events related to cardiovascular disease.

8.1 Introduction

Cardiovascular disease along with stroke is the leading cause of death. The basis of cardiovascular disease is the impairment of the endothelial wall followed by inflammation of the wall leading to the formation of atherosclerosis further causing the myocardial infarction and stroke. The major risk factors are hypertension, obesity, and diabetes [1].

8.2 Molecular Imaging

Molecular Imaging is the noninvasive visualization, characterization, and quantification of biological processes at the molecular and subcellular levels. It has the important role in understanding the biology, early detection, accurate diagnosis, and monitoring response to the therapy. There are a lot of advancements seen in the imaging modalities for the evaluation of cardiovascular disease. Previously PET

S. Shaikh, *PET-CT in Infection and Inflammation*,
https://doi.org/10.1007/978-981-15-9801-2_8

was the important imaging modality but with the advent of PET-CT and PET-MR, a lot of newer applications are being used. In relation to cardiovascular disease, PET-CT is useful in evaluating coronary vasculature in myocardium, cardiac amyloidosis, cardiac Sarcoidosis, cerebrovascular disease, acute aortic syndrome, and cardiac and vascular neoplasms, cardiac and vascular infections [2]. 3D PET-CT is also important for the better resolution of the myocardial perfusion imaging, which will reduce the time of the imaging protocols, reduce radiation exposure, and increased applications in cerebrovascular disease.

8.3   Normal Cardiac Anatomy

The heart's main source of energy is the fatty acids with 70% of adenosine triphosphate is derived from the fatty acid oxidation. The remaining energy sources are glucose, lactate, and ketone. Under the influence of the stress, pathology, and various insults, the ratio of dependence on various substrates changes and the ultimate response will be based on these factors. In certain conditions like diabetes, the amount of uptake in myocardium is less thus increasing the load on fatty acid metabolism. Normal cardiac anatomy consists of endocardium, myocardium, epicardium, and pericardium. The right atrium receives venous drainage from the body and right ventricle pumps the blood to the lungs for oxygenation. After this, oxygenated blood enters the left atrium and again pumped into the left ventricle. The arterial supply of the heart is from the right coronary artery and left main coronary artery. The LM branch into the left LAD and left circumflex artery. Then the right coronary artery supplies blood to the left ventricle in inferior aspect. LAD supplies blood to anterior aspect of the left ventricle and septum. The left circumflex artery supplies blood to the lateral and posterior left ventricle [3].

8.4   Cardiac Imaging Techniques

8.4.1   Myocardial Perfusion Imaging

Myocardial perfusion imaging is indicated for known or suspected cases of coronary artery disease. The radiotracers used for cardiac perfusion imaging are 82-Rb and 13-N-Ammonia. However, the half-life of both these radiotracers is different. 13-9-Ammonia needs on-site cyclotron. The myocardial perfusion imaging can also be done SPECT myocardial imaging. But PET myocardial perfusion imaging is master having superior attenuation correction and higher spatial and temporal resolution. 18F-based radiotracers may have a longer half-life compared with the radiotracers used for cardiac perfusion (Fig. 8.1).

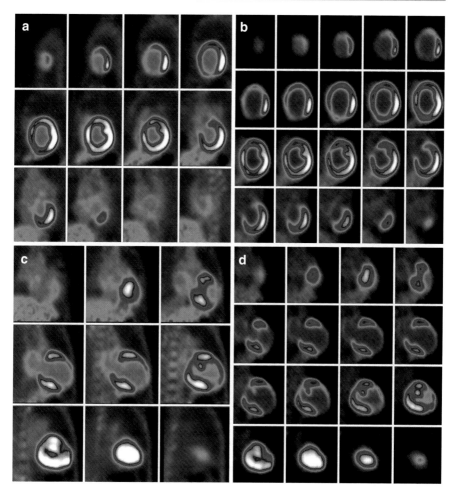

Fig. 8.1 FDG PET showing dilated left ventricular cavity. Reduced tracer uptake in apex, anterior, apical septal, apical inferior, and mid-inferior walls

8.4.2   Cardiac Viability Imaging

Cardiac viability imaging is the imaging of the myocardium, especially in cases of suspected patients. FDG is also preferred because of high spatial resolution and accuracy. With this, the viable tissue in the area of perfusion defect in the previous study. This is an area where FDG uptake corresponds to viability scan.

8.4.3   Normal Vascular Anatomy (Non-coronary)

The left ventricle ejects the blood into the systemic circulation via the aorta. This aorta branches into bigger and eventually smaller arteries. The perfusion happens at the level of capillaries, where the blood is returning via the venous system.

All the arteries are composed of three layers. The outer layer is adventitia, media is the middle layer, and intima is the inner layer. Atherosclerosis apex the intimal layer while other cardiovascular pathologies can affect the other two layers.

8.4.4   Coronary Vascular Imaging

FDG PET evaluates coronary vascularity by the perfusion imaging. Additional advantage is to evaluate the cause of pathologies involving the vasculature.

8.5   Imaging Protocols

8.5.1   Myocardial Perfusion

Myocardial perfusion imaging is indicated for patients with known or suspected coronary artery disease. Radiotracer used are 82-Rb and 13-N-Ammonia. Patient preparation overnight fasting, avoid caffeine-containing food products for 24 h and Theophylline-containing medicines for 48 h. Rest and stress images are acquired on different days. First rest images are acquired and in 2-day studies stress images are acquired first. Scout view of cardiac is taken that confirmed the field of view. Standard cardiac imaging view starts from lung apices to the base of the heart. Radiotracer (Rb-82) should be injected. After injection, an emission scan typically starts around 5 min and should be obtained. ECG lead is placed to evaluate the cardiac status. In this scan, continuous monitoring of the patient with ECG, blood pressure, and heart rate is important [4–7] (Figs. 8.2 and 8.3).

8.5.2   Cardiac Viability

Cardiac viability imaging is usually advised for the suspected high-risk cardiac patients who have a fair chance of revascularization and there is a suspicion of hibernating myocardium. Contraindications are the routine contraindications for PET scan. Patients with diabetes or insulin should continue their medications and dietic precautions. On arrival of the patient, blood glucose is checked and insulin administration can be done under the guidance of the referring physician [8, 9].

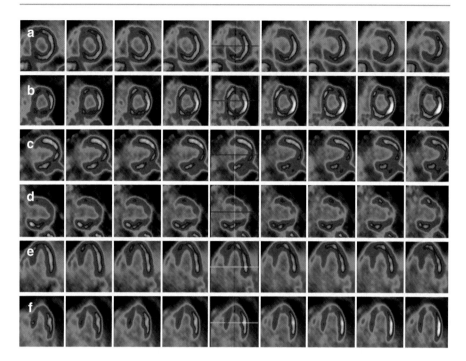

Fig. 8.2 Ammonia scan showing viable myocardium in the entire septal wall. Rest all walls show normal perfusion and dilated left ventricular cavity

8.6 Cardiac Pathologies

8.6.1 Cardiac Sarcoidosis

Cardiac sarcoidosis protocol is used for patients suspected of sarcoidosis. The patient preparation is same as mentioned in the above paragraph. In cases, if glucose level is acceptable 10 mci FDG PET radiotracer administered and sarcoid protocol scan is done. This protocol is more focussed for evalaution of Sarcoidosis in known or suspected cases [10–14].

8.6.2 Cardiac Amyloidosis

FDG PET has shown significant results in the evaluation of amyloid plaques [15–17]. With these optimal technical parameters should be used for evaluation.

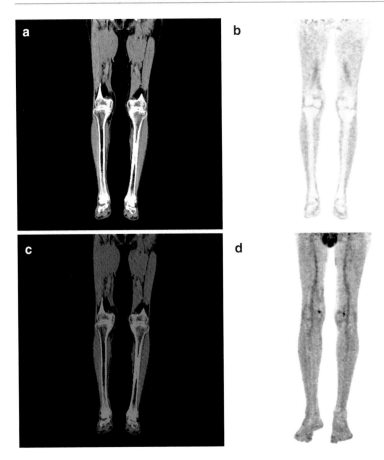

Fig. 8.3 Lower limb FDG PET-CT showing diffuse irregular linear mild uptake in PET images (**b**, **d**) and fused image (**c**) with SUV max of 2 along the bilateral superficial femoral and popliteal arteries suggestive of atheromatous changes. CT image does not show any significant changes

8.7   Cardiovascular Infection, Inflammation, and Neoplasm

Whole-body FDG PET-CT is the commonest and widely used protocol to evaluate malignancy. But nowadays with the advent of other applications, infection and inflammation are also commonly being used for the whole body applications. The same criteria of the routine whole-body PET protocol is being used [18–20].

8.7.1   Pathology and Imaging Findings

8.7.2   Cardiac/Pericardiac Imaging

8.8 Perfusion Scan

Normal myocardial perfusion in the rest state shows diffuse uptake in the entire myocardium. Any focal perfusion defect signifies the myocardial infarction or any artifact. A stress myocardial perfusion scan is done after injecting the radiotracer to see any focal defects. A normal stress scan with no perfusion defects signifies the normal coronary arteries. This quantification of perfusion defect in the various myocardial walls signifies the vessel that is involved, for example, perfusion defect in the inferior wall suggests right coronary artery narrowing. The perfusion defect in the anterior wall or septum or apex shows LAD narrowing. The perfusion defect in the anterolateral or inferolateral wall of the myocardium suggests the left circumflex narrowing [21, 22].

8.9 Viability Scan

Viability shows the amount of normal viable tissue on FDG. This is based on the fixed defect in the perfusion imaging. The evaluation of scar/infarct does not show FDG activity that shows focal defect on perfusion imaging [23, 24].

8.10 Nonischemic Cardiomyopathies and Inflammatory Disorders

8.10.1 Sarcoidosis

Sarcoidosis is a granulomatous disease with noncaseating granulomas and involves the multiorgan system. The cardiac manifestation is in the form of cardiomyopathies or arrhythmias. In one of the studies, 25% of patients with sarcoidosis shows cardiac involvement [25, 26]. Sarcoidosis also involves the pericardium, myocardium, and endocardium of the atrium or ventricle. The left lateral wall is the commonest wall and involving all the walls. The common is the basal septum which involves the conducting system. Myocardial involvement resembles in a very patchy way inflammation and granulomas can involve the myocardial walls with associated inflammation. PET-CT shows the uptake corresponding to the pathologies. Sarcoid imaging also evaluates the defect on resting scan and stress scan depending on the amount of inflammation and associated ischemia or infarct. Thus, on this basis, PET shows a significant role in diagnosing as well as assessing the treatment response.

8.10.2 Nonischemic Inflammatory Cardiomyopathy

As already discussed, PET-CT has an important role in the evaluation of ischemic changes in this entity. Now, it also plays important role in the evaluation of nonischemic inflammatory cardiomyopathies, inflammatory myocarditis, myocardial stress evaluation, or Takotsubo cardiomyopathy. The mechanism of Takotsubo cardiomyopathy is unknown but is related to increased catecholamine levels and stress induced, neuropeptides which can cause vascular spasm or myosite injury [27–29].

8.10.3 Amyloidosis

It is caused by abnormal deposits of amyloid plaques [30]. The amyloidosis is also seen in the form of amyloid plaques in suspected Alzheimer's disease. 18F NaF PET also plays important role in subcategorizing transthyretin-related cardiac amyloid vs. light-chain cardiac amyloidosis.

8.10.4 Infection

Recent studies have shown the ability of PET to diagnose prosthetic valve infection and infection of implanted electronic devices [31, 32]. PET shows significant endocarditis and the same analysis to evaluate infective myocarditis.

8.11 Vascular Imaging

8.11.1 Atherosclerosis

Atherosclerotic plaque can be associated with myocardial metabolism due to the altered coronary blood flow. PET shows the assessment of atherosclerotic plaque and important entity and is associated with inflammation [33, 34]. Atherosclerotic process may also have inflammation and calcification depending on the pathophysiological process of the disease. PET also plays an important role in the evaluation of monitoring response to the treatment of atherosclerosis. The FDG uptake in the pre- and post-therapy signifies the treatment response.

8.11.2 Aneurysm

Aneurysm is most commonly seen in the aorta. The FDG uptake is associated with the amount of inflammation and macrophage accumulation. Any aneurysmal change in the form of pain, rupture, or stable aneurysm signifies the more benign course [35].

8.11.3 Coarctation of Aorta, Aortic Dissection, and Intramural Hematoma

Coarctation of aorta also can show mild uptake if associated with the inflammation. Aortic dissection can be acute or chronic. The FDG uptake is also seen in the

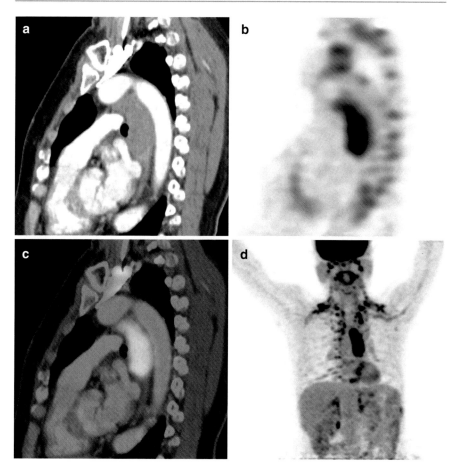

Fig. 8.4 CT image (**a**) showing focal narrowing of the posterior aspect of arch of aorta suggestive of coarctation of aorta with no FDG uptake. PET (**b, d**) and fused images (**c**) shows no uptake

intramural region where the platelets adhere to leukocytes. This focal area shows corresponding FDG uptake [36, 37] (Fig. 8.4).

Vasculitis
The role of FDG PET-CT is significantly explained in a separate chapter.

8.12 Cerebrovascular Disease

The cerebrovascular disease is again an important entity with a lot of morbidity and mortality. PET-CT can be used to evaluate the cause of cerebrovascular disease, ischemic penumbra to evaluate the planning. Inflammation is one of the important causes of cerebrovascular disease [38, 39].

8.13   Graft Infection

PET-CT plays an important role in the evaluation of vascular graft infections, which is not evaluated by any other imaging modalities. This infection is proportional to the amount of infection, inflammation, and complications [40–42].

Infection due to Vascular Pathologies
Few of the vascular pathologies will show significant pathological changes. One of the common pathology is diabetic involvement like diabetic foot where significant stenosis, soft tissue swelling, bony erosion, and destructions. Many other pathologies related to vascular involvement will also show significant changes in the PET-CT (Figs. 8.5, 8.6, and 8.7).

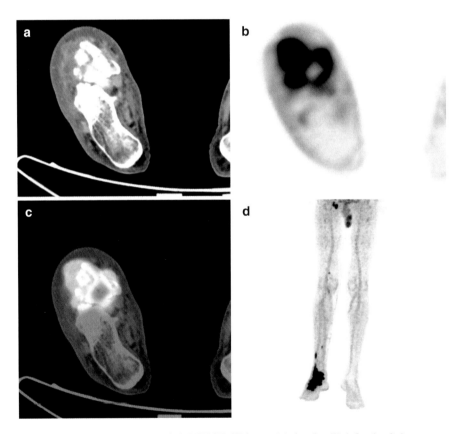

Fig. 8.5 Known diabetic. Lower limb PET-CT, CT image (**a**) showing ill-defined soft tissue component involving the right ankle and foot with erosion and destruction of the tarsal bone and associated soft tissue swelling. This soft tissue shows significant uptake in PET (**b, d**) and fused images (**c**) management with SUV max of 8.2

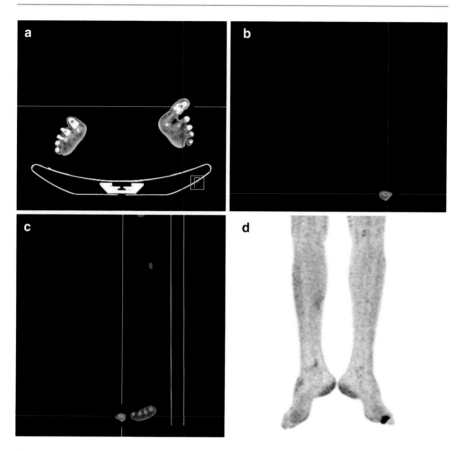

Fig. 8.6 Lower limbs FDG PET-CT showing small nodular thickening on CT (**a**) and nodular uptake in great toe and left foot on PET images (**b, d**) and fused image (**c**). No history of diabetes. On examination of ulcerative lesion this findings are suggestive of nonhealing ulcer

Fig. 8.7 Fused PET-CT image of the Fig. 8.6 showing mild nodular uptake of SUV max 3.1 suggestive of nonhealing ulcer

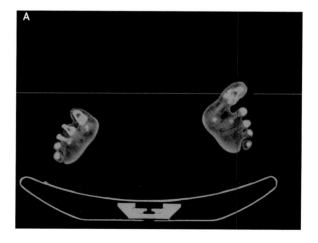

8.14   Hibernating Myocardium

In the suspected hibernating myocardium, the revascularizing process, criteria to diagnosis viable tissue on FDG PET.

8.15   Summary

Thus, PET-CT is an important modality for the evaluation of a variety of inflammatory infective disorders in cardiovascular diseases. PET is significantly useful in all the conditions mentioned above. Newer radiotracers and newer techniques will show promising results in diagnosing and monitoring the response to treatment in a variety of diseases.

References

1. Murillo H, Restrepo CS, Marmol-Velez JA, et al. Infectious diseases of the heart: pathophysiology, clinical and imaging overview. Radiographics. 2016;36:963–83.
2. Brunken RC. Promising new 18F-labeled tracers for PET myocardial perfusion imaging. J Nucl Med. 2015;56(10):1478–9.
3. Buckberg GD. Basic science review: the helix and the heart. J Thorac Cardiovasc Surg. 2002;124:863–83. https://doi.org/10.1067/mtc.2002.122439.
4. Rieber J, Huber A, Erhard I, Mueller S, Schweyer M, Koenig A, Schiele TM, Theisen K, Siebert U, Schoenberg SO, Reiser M, Klauss V. Cardiac magnetic resonance perfusion imaging for the functional assessment of coronary artery disease: a comparison with coronary angiography and fractional flow reserve. Eur Heart J. 2006;27:1465–71.
5. Thomson LEJ, Kim RJ, Judd RM. Magnetic resonance imaging for the assessment of myocardial viability. J Magn Reson Imaging. 2004;19(6):771–88. https://doi.org/10.1002/jmri.20075.
6. Brazier J, Hottenrott C, Buckberg G. Non-coronary collateral myocardial blood flow. Ann Thorac Surg. 1975;19:426–35.
7. Pascual TN, Mercuri M, El-Haj N, Bom HH, Lele V, Al-Mallah MH, et al. Nuclear cardiology practice in Asia: analysis of radiation exposure and best practice for myocardial perfusion imaging - results from the IAEA Nuclear Cardiology Protocols Cross-Sectional Study (INCAPS). Circ J. 2017;81(4):501–10.
8. Henzlova MJ, Duvall WL, Einstein AJ, Travin MI, Verberne HJ. ASNC imaging guidelines for SPECT nuclear cardiology procedures: stress, protocols, and tracers. J Nucl Cardiol. 2016;23(3):606–39.
9. Malik D, Basher R, Vadi S, et al. Cardiac metastasis from lung cancer mimicking as perfusion defect on N-13 ammonia and FDG myocardial viability PET/CT scan. J Nucl Cardiol. 2016; https://doi.org/10.1007/s12350-016-0609-x.
10. Skali H, Schulman AR, Dorbala S. 18F-FDGPET/CT for the assessment of myocardial sarcoidosis. Curr Cardiol Rep. 2013;15(4):352.
11. Okumura W, Iwasaki T, Toyama T, et al. Usefulness of fasting 18F-FDG PET in identification of cardiac sarcoidosis. J Nucl Med. 2004;45(12):1989–98.
12. Miller CT, Sweiss NJ, Lu Y. FDGPET/CT evidence of effective treatment of cardiac sarcoidosis with Adalimumab. Clin Nucl Med. 2016;41(5):417–8.
13. Lapa C, Reiter T, Kircher M, et al. Somatostat in receptor based PET/CT in patients with the suspicion of cardiac sarcoidosis: an initial comparison to cardiac MRI. Oncotarget. 2016;7(47):77807–14.

14. Lhommel R, Sempoux C, Ivanoiu A, et al. Is 18F-flutemetamol PET/CT able to reveal cardiac amyloidosis? Clin Nucl Med. 2014;39(8):747–9.
15. Garcia-Gonzalez P, Cozar-Santiago MD, Maceira AM. Cardiac amyloidosis detected using 18F-florbetapir PET/CT. Rev Esp Cardiol (Engl Ed). 2016;69(12):1215.
16. Gagliardi C, Tabacchi E, Bonfiglioli R, et al. Does the etiology of cardiac amyloidosis determine the myocardial uptake of [18F]-NaFPET/CT? J Nucl Cardiol. 2017;24(2):746–9.
17. Li JS, Sexton DJ, Mick N, et al. Proposed modifications to the Duke criteria for the diagnosis of infective endocarditis. Clin Infect Dis. 2000;30:633–8.
18. Baddour LM, Wilson WR, Bayer AS, et al. Infective endocarditis in adults: diagnosis, antimicrobial therapy, and management of complications: a scientific statement for healthcare professionals from the American Heart Association. Circulation. 2015;132:1435–86.
19. Gomes A, Glaudemans AWJM, Touw DJ, et al. Diagnostic value of imaging in infective endocarditis: a systematic review. Lancet Infect Dis. 2017;17:e1–14.
20. Otsuka R, Kubo N, Miyazaki Y, Kawahara M, Takaesu J, Fukuchi K. Current status of stress myocardial perfusion imaging pharmaceuticals and radiation exposure in Japan: results from a nationwide survey. J Nucl Cardiol. 2017;24(6):1850–5.
21. Xue H, Hansen MS, Nielles-vallespin S, Arai AE, Kellman P. Inline quantitative myocardial perfusion flow mapping. JCMR/ISMRM Work. 2016;18:4–6.
22. Gewirtz H, Dilsizian V. Myocardial viability: survival mechanisms and molecular imaging targets in acute and chronic ischemia. Circ Res. 2017;120:1197–212.
23. Packard RR, Huang SC, Dahlbom M, Czernin J, Maddahi J. Absolute quantitation of myocardial blood flow in human subjects with or without myocardial ischemia using dynamic flurpiridaz F 18 PET. J Nucl Med. 2014;55:1438–44. https://doi.org/10.2967/jnumed.114.141093.
24. Murtagh G, Laffin LJ, Beshai JF, Maffessanti F, Bonham CA, Patel AV, Yu Z, Addetia K, Mor-Avi V, Moss JD, Hogarth DK, Sweiss NJ, Lang RM, Patel AR. Prognosis of myocardial damage in sarcoidosis patients with preserved left ventricular ejection fraction: risk stratification using cardiovascular magnetic resonance. Circ Cardiovasc Imaging. 2016;9:e003738.
25. Vita T, Okada DR, Veillet-Chowdhury M, Bravo PE, Mullins E, Hulten E, Agrawal M, Madan R, Taqueti VR, Steigner M, Skali H, Kwong RY, Stewart GC, Dorbala S, Di Carli MF, Blankstein R. Complementary value of cardiac magnetic resonance imaging and positron emission tomography/computed tomography in the assessment of cardiac sarcoidosis. Circ Cardiovasc Imaging. 2018;11:e007030.
26. Vrtovec B, Poglajen G, Lezaic L, Sever M, Domanovic D, Cernelc P, Socan A, Schrepfer S, Torre-Amione G, Haddad F, Wu JC. Effects of intracoronary CD34+ stem cell transplantation in nonischemic dilated cardiomyopathy patients: 5-year follow-up. Circ Res. 2013;112:165–73. https://doi.org/10.1161/CIRCRESAHA.112.276519.
27. Hare JM, DiFede DL, Rieger AC, et al. Randomized comparison of allogeneic versus autologous mesenchymal stem cells for non-ischemic dilated cardiomyopathy: POSEIDON-DCM trial. J Am Coll Cardiol. 2017;69:526–37. https://doi.org/10.1016/j.jacc.2016.11.009.
28. Namdar M, Rager O, Priamo J, Frei A, Noble S, Amzalag G, Ratib O, Nkoulou R. Prognostic value of revascularising viable myocardium in elderly patients with stable coronary artery disease and left ventricular dysfunction: a PET/CT study. Int J Cardiovasc Imaging. 2018; https://doi.org/10.1007/s10554-018-1380-7.
29. Morgenstern R, Yeh R, Castano A, Maurer MS, Bokhari S. 18Fluorine sodium fluoride positron emission tomography, a potential biomarker of transthyretin cardiac amyloidosis. J Nucl Cardiol. 2017; https://doi.org/10.1007/s12350-017-0799-x.
30. Millar B, Moore J, Mallon P, et al. Molecular diagnosis of infective endocarditis: a new Duke's criterion. Scand J Infect Dis. 2001;33:673–80.
31. Swart LE, Gomes A, Scholtens AM, et al. Improving the diagnostic performance of 18F-FDG PET/CT in prosthetic heart valve endocarditis. Circulation. 2018;138:1412–27.
32. Bala G, Blykers A, Xavier C, et al. Targeting of vascular cell adhesion molecule-1 by 18F-labelled nanobodies for PET/CT imaging of inflamed atherosclerotic plaques. Eur Heart J Cardiovasc Imaging. 2016;17(9):1001–8.

33. Tahara N, Kai H, Ishibashi M, et al. Simvastatin attenuates plaque inflammation: evaluation by fluorodeoxyglucose positron emission tomography. J Am Coll Cardiol. 2006;48(9):1825–31.
34. Courtois A, Nusgens BV, Hustinx R, Namur G, Gomez P, Somja J, et al. 18F-FDG uptake assessed by PET/CT in abdominal aortic aneurysms is associated with cellular and molecular alterations prefacing wall deterioration and rupture. J Nucl Med. 2013;54:1740–7.
35. Marini C, Morbelli S, Armonino R, Spinella G, Riondato M, Massollo M, et al. Direct relationship between cell density and FDG uptake in asymptomatic aortic aneurysm close to surgical threshold: an in vivo and in vitro study. Eur J Nucl Med Mol Imaging. 2012;39:91–101.
36. Tahara N, Hirakata S, Okabe K, Tahara A, Honda A, Igata S, et al. FDG-PET/CT images during 5 years before acute aortic dissection. Eur Heart J. 2016;37:1933.
37. Yang F, Luo J, Hou Q, Xie N, Nie Z, Huang W, et al. Predictive value of 18F-FDG PET/CT in patients with acute type B aortic intramural hematoma. J Nucl Cardiol. 2017; https://doi.org/10.1007/s12350-017-1014-9.
38. Bartels S, Kyavar L, Blumstein N, et al. FDG PET findings leading to the diagnosis of neurosarcoidosis. Clin Neurol Neurosurg. 2013;115(1):85–8.
39. Kampe KKW, Roetermund R, Tienken M, et al. Diagnostic value of positron emission tomography combined with computed tomography for evaluating critically ill neurological patients. Front Neurol. 2017;8:33.
40. Sah BR, Husmann L, Mayer D, et al. Diagnostic performance of 18F-FDG-PET/CT in vascular graft infections. Eur J Vasc Endovasc Surg. 2015;49(4):455–64.
41. Husmann L, Sah BR, Scherrer A, et al. ^{18}F-FDG PET/CT for therapy control in vascular graft infections: a first feasibility study. J Nucl Med. 2015;56(7):1024–9.
42. Sarikaya I, Elgazzar AH, Alfeeli MA, Sharma PN, Sarikaya A. Status of F-18 fluorodeoxyglucose uptake in normal and hibernating myocardium after glucose and insulin loading. J Saudi Heart Assoc. 2018;30:75–85.

PET-CT in Peripheral Vascular Pathologies

9

Key Points

Peripheral vascular inflammation is one of the important causes of cardiovascular disease. FDG PET is used for quantification of the metabolic uptake by the principle of the molecular biomarker.

The metabolically active macrophages add as pro-inflammatory in the rupture-prone atherosclerotic plaque.

18F FDG PET is used to detect arterial inflammation and early atherosclerosis. Thus, cardiovascular risk is evaluated.

9.1 Introduction

Atherosclerosis is an inflammatory disease of the inner wall of the large and medium-size arteries. A couple of factors, which impact atherosclerosis, are based on the involvement of the disease, degree of the blood flow obstruction, and associated predisposing factors [1, 2]. With the available imaging modalities, the imaging of atherosclerosis is well established.

9.2 Pathogenesis of Atherosclerosis

Atherosclerosis is initiated by a series of pro-inflammatory events that are due to endothelial disruption, macrophage activation, infiltration, lipid accumulation, and ultimately plaque formation [3, 4]. The vascular plaques are the hallmark and predictive biomarker for developing the risk in vessels. However, all biomarkers are not consistent to evaluate the risk potential for thrombosis resulting in infarct or stroke. One of the important examples is chronic low-grade inflammation associated with

© The Author(s), under exclusive license to Springer Nature
Singapore Pte Ltd. 2021
S. Shaikh, *PET-CT in Infection and Inflammation*,
https://doi.org/10.1007/978-981-15-9801-2_9

the immune response to HIV infection and cardiovascular disease. However, the inflammation and its biomarkers in the form of D-dimer, cytokines, which are neither specific nor sensitive are still being used.

9.3   Role of FDG PET-CT

The use of 18 FDG uptake by macrophages in the arterial wall acts as noninvasive, sensitive, and specific for early atheroma formation. The role of PET-CT is to detect the uptake in macrophages and to quantify associated inflammation in atherosclerosis and in vulnerable plaques. One of the pilot studies has shown diffuse inflammation in the carotid and aortic valves in the patients of mild cardiovascular disease risk [5, 6]. FDG PET-CT is also used to monitor the amount of atherogenesis by various associated factors. One of the important criteria for carotid artery Doppler is a carotid artery intima-media thickness that is usually measured in B-mode images and their assessment can be done by focal wall thickening and diffuse wall thickening. Technically PET-CT was done to evaluate the high-resolution vessel wall quantification for early atheromatous changes. FDG PET is based on the quantification of uptake along the walls of the vessel wall. This provides optimal co-registration. This PET-CT findings are consistent with the associated Doppler findings like focal atheromatous changes with uptake. Other parameters to be measured in the suspected high-risk patients are the lipid profile, especially triglycerides and LDL cholesterol levels. The FDG PET-CT can differentiate between associated early atherosclerosis and early vascular inflammation based on the FDG uptake. In early atherosclerosis, the FDG uptake is not significant, however, in vascular inflammations depending on the acuteness, the amount of uptake is proportionate to it [7, 8] (Figs. 9.1 and 9.2).

9.4   Vascular Inflammation

Comparatively, vascular inflammation is more predisposing to the incidence of myocardial infarction and stroke. However, this suggestion is based on the associated circulating pro-inflammatory or pro-oxidant biomarkers. This vascular inflammation is more prominent in the high-risk cases and inflammations like immune-compromised infection. Thus, FDG is significantly important to quantify the pro-inflammatory events that are biochemically related to atherogenesis [9–12]. And these biochemical events are important for guiding the amount of risk. Thus, FDG PET can detect early low-level vascular inflammation in people with HIV. Dual point imaging is also important for the evaluation.

The retention index percentage was calculated by subtracting the SUVmax in early images from the SUVmax in delayed images and dividing by SUVmax in early images [13, 14].

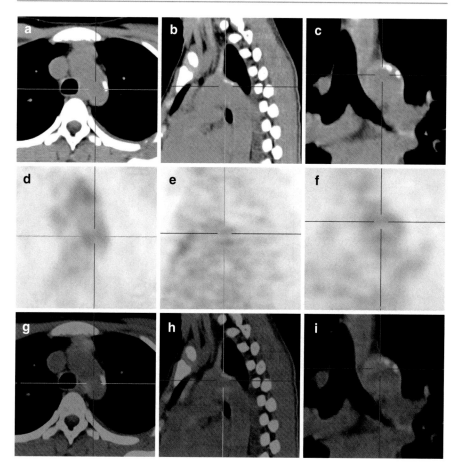

Fig. 9.1 Limited PET-CT chest, CT image (**a–c**) showing small atheromatous calcification subtle mild uptake along the arch of aorta with associated atheromatous small calcifications in PET (**d, f**) and fused images (**g–i**). SUV max 1.8

(SUVmax in delayed images—SUVmax in early images) SUVmax in early images (SUVmax in delayed images—SUVmax in early images) SUVmax in early images.

The FDG uptake by the aortic arterial wall in the delayed images was graded as follows:

• Grade 1 when arterial FDG activity is equal or less than the blood pool FDG activity.
• Grade 2 when arterial FDG activity is higher than the blood pool FDG activity but less than that of the liver.
• Grade 3 when arterial FDG activity is higher than the blood pool but equal to the liver FDG activity.

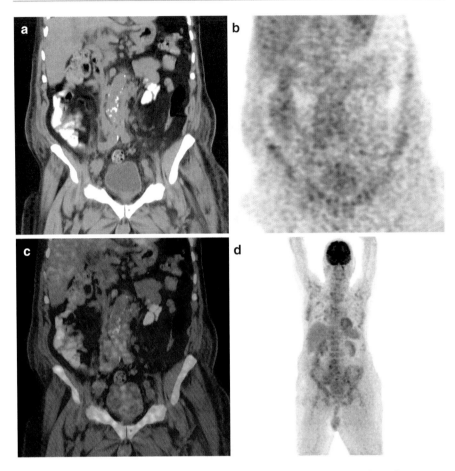

Fig. 9.2 Whole-body PET-CT with abdominal sections, CT image (**a**) showing atheromatous changes in abdominal aorta with small calcifications in PET images (**c, d**) and fused images (**b**) with no FDG uptake

- Grade 4 when arterial FDG activity is higher than the blood pool and slightly higher to the liver FDG activity.

Aortic arterial wall comprises of four parts of the aorta, ascending aorta, aortic arch, descending thoracic aorta, and descending abdominal aorta. Within each part intimal HU mean, maximum intimal thickness, degree of intimal changes, degree of aortic calcification, and intraluminal diameter are the parameters for the evaluation of the vessel wall.

Intimal HU mean were measured in non-enhanced images by multiple drawing regions of interest including the aortic wall measuring HU mean in each drawing. Then the mean of all readings were calculated for each part.

Intimal thickness is measured in the post-contrast images to differentiate the enhanced luminal blood from the relatively less enhancing aortic wall. The severity of intimal changes was shown by a percentage of thickenings of the circumference of the aortic wall for each segment. The intimal changes were evaluated qualitatively including outline irregularity with or without calcific changes. Regarding intraluminal diameter, the internal luminal diameter is measured in the largest cross-section of the aortic diameter except in the aortic arch where the shortest axis is used. The ratio of the aortic diameter to body surface area was used to know the differences in individual body build. The degree of aortic calcification was measured in non-enhanced CT images. It was expressed in the form of a percentage of the longitudinal dimensions of each length.

9.5   Venous Thromboembolic Disease

Venous thromboembolism is one of the common clinical entities comprising deep vein thrombosis and pulmonary embolism. The early diagnosis is challenging because of nonspecific clinical presentation, which may result in a fatal disease. The conventional imaging modalities have several pitfalls. Whole-body FDG PET is having promising results due to inflammation and thrombosis, which are interlinked pathogenesis wise. Demonstration of DVT and pulmonary embolism by FDG PET are easily FDG avid. Another advantage of FDG PET is to analyze the cause of DVT and PE, especially in malignant settings. Whole-body FDG PET-CT provides an important screening to identify the morphology and cause of the thrombus [13, 15]. This can be done by the quantifiying the amount of metabolic activity that shows the cause of DVT and PE as malignant or non-malignant. With this PET-CT is emerging as the important imaging modality to diagnose venous thromboembolism its extent cause, characterization-associated complications, and response to therapy. The response to therapy is evaluated after the particular dose and regimen for that particular disease is administered and rescan after completion of the therapy. Most importantly FDG PET determines whether the thrombus is active, chronic, or inactive (Figs. 9.3, 9.4, 9.5, 9.6, and 9.7).

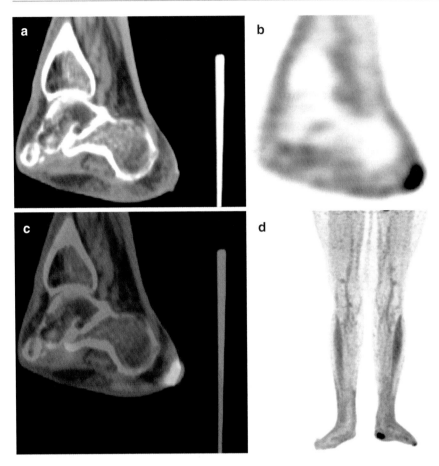

Fig. 9.3 Focal area of nodular soft tissue lesion on CT image (**a**) at the posterior aspect of the heel with associated subcutaneous edema and PET uptake of 6.7 in PET image (**b**, **c**) and fused image suggestive of inflammatory lesion. Prominent uptake bilateral gastrocnemius muscles suggest no relevance

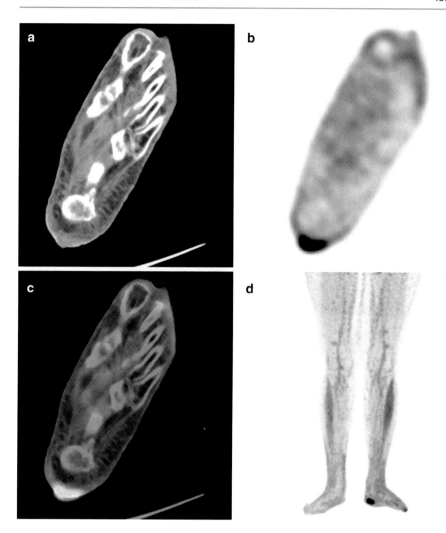

Fig. 9.4 Limited PET-CT both lower limbs, CT image (**a**) showing nodular soft tissue lesion with skin ulceration and PET images (**b**, **d**) and fused image (**c**) showing significant FDG uptake with SUV max of 6.6. Histopathologically suggestive of inflammatory lesion

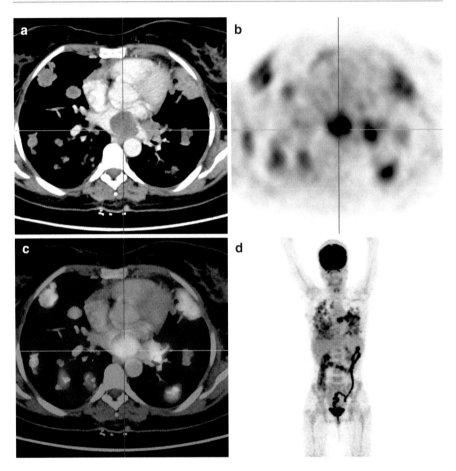

Fig. 9.5 Whole-body PET-CT with multiple lung metastases (**a**) showing mild uptake in the rounded lesion in the left atrium in fused (**c**) and PET images (**b, d**) with SUV max of 6.4 consistent with inactive intraluminal thrombus

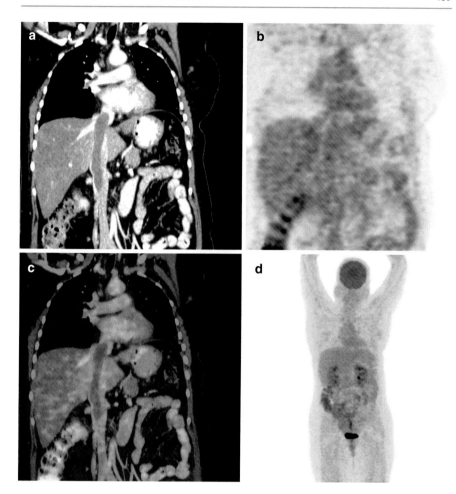

Fig. 9.6 Whole-body PET-CT with upper abdominal sections showing linear irregular nonactive intraluminal thrombus in the IVC in CT image (**a**) with no metabolic activity in (**b–d**) images

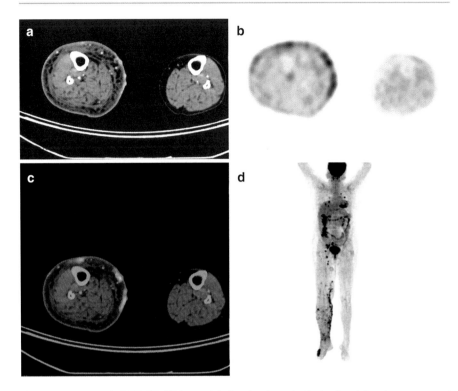

Fig. 9.7 Whole-body PET-CT CT image (**a**) showing irregular lesion involving the caecum and ascending colon with nodes in the right external iliac region. PET images (**b, d**) and fused images (**c**) showing with a significant amount of uptake SUV max of 6.2. The right lower limb is bulky with subcutaneous edema and nodular skin thickening. Right proximal posterior tibial vein shows intraluminal thrombus on CT with mild tracer activity SUV max of 4.0 suggestive of deep vein thrombosis in right lower limb

References

1. Montecucco F, Mach F. Atherosclerosis is an inflammatory disease. Semin Immunopathol. 2009;31:1–3.
2. Ferrari E, Vidal R, Chevallier T, et al. Atherosclerosis of the thoracic aorta and aortic debris as a marker of poor prognosis: benefit of oral anticoagulants. J Am Coll Cardiol. 1999;33(5):1317–22.
3. Sakakura K, Nakano M, Otsuka F, Ladich E, Kolodgie FD, Virmani R. Pathophysiology of atherosclerosis plaque progression. Heart Lung Circ. 2013;22(6):399–411.
4. Tarkin JM, Dweck MR, Evans NR, et al. Imaging atherosclerosis. Circ Res. 2016;118(4):750–69.
5. Cavalcanti Filho JLG, Ronaldo de Souza Leão L, Luiz de Souza Machado N, et al. PET/CT and vascular disease: current concepts. Eur J Radiol. 2011;80(1):60–7.
6. Virmani R, Kolodgie FD, Burke AP, et al. Atherosclerotic plaque progression and vulnerability to rupture: angiogenesis as a source of intra-plaque hemorrhage. Arterioscler Thromb Vasc Biol. 2005;25(10):2054–61.
7. Cybulsky MI, Iiyama K, Li H, et al. A major role for VCAM-1, but not ICAM-1, in early atherosclerosis. J Clin Invest. 2001;107(10):1255–62.

8. Tatsumi M, Cohade C, Nakamoto Y, et al. Fluorodeoxyglucose uptake in the aortic wall at PET/CT: possible finding for active atherosclerosis. Radiology. 2003;229(3):831–7.

9. Meirelles GSP, Gonen M, Strauss HW. 18F-FDG uptake and calcifications in the thoracic aorta on positron emission tomography/computed tomography examinations: frequency and stability on serial scans. J Thorac Imaging. 2011;26(1):54–62.

10. Rudd JH, Myers KS, Bansilal S, et al. Relationships among regional arterial inflammation, calcification, risk factors, and biomarkers: a prospective fluorodeoxyglucose positron-emission tomography/computed tomography imaging study. Circulation. 2009;2(2):107–15.

11. Tawakol A, Migrino RQ, Bashian GG, et al. In vivo 18Ffluorodeoxyglucose positron emission tomography imaging provides a non-invasive measure of carotid plaque inflammation in patients. J Am Coll Cardiol. 2006;48:1818–24.

12. Evans NR, Tarkin JM, Chowdhury MM, et al. PET imaging of atherosclerotic disease: advancing plaque assessment from anatomy to pathophysiology. Curr Atheroscler Rep. 2016;18:30.

13. Tawakol A, Migrino RQ, Bashian GG, et al. In vivo 18F-fluorodeoxyglucose positron emission tomography imaging provides a noninvasive measure of carotid plaque inflammation in patients. J Am Coll Cardiol. 2006;48(9):1818–24. https://doi.org/10.1016/j.jacc.2006.05.076.

14. Puchner SB, Liu T, Mayrhofer T, et al. High-risk plaque detected on coronary CT angiography predicts acute coronary syndromes independent of significant stenosis in acute chest pain: results from the ROMICAT-II trial. J Am Coll Cardiol. 2014;64(7):684–92. https://doi.org/10.1016/j.jacc.2014.05.039.

15. Figueroa AL, Subramanian SS, Cury RC, et al. Distribution of inflammation within carotid atherosclerotic plaques with high-risk morphological features: a comparison between positron emission tomography activity, plaque morphology, and histopathology. Circ Cardiovasc Imaging. 2012;5(1):69–77. https://doi.org/10.1161/CIRCIMAGING.110.959478.

PET-CT in Vasculitis

10

Key Points

Vasculitis is the inflammation of vessels that can be a large vessel, medium vessel, and small vessel. The evaluation of vasculitis is very crucial for timely and accurate diagnosis. Till now the temporal artery biopsy was only the confirmatory but with the rapid growth of technological advances many newer modalities with wider applications are coming up. PET-CT is now the most advanced available imaging modality and is being commonly used for the diagnosis of vasculitis. Another subset of the applications is the clinical findings like headache, demographic features like age, and ESR. The various inflammatory markers are being used but are non-specific and not concurrent with the final diagnosis.

10.1 Introduction

Vasculitis is the inflammation of the vessel wall. Diagnosis of vasculitis is a big challenge when vasculitis is affecting the vital organs and the presenting with non-specific symptoms. The diagnosis of this is exceedingly difficult and cannot be made out with good sensitivity with the available conventional imaging modalities. Till date temporal artery biopsy was considered as a gold standard but getting the optimal biopsy is difficult. With recent technological developments, ^{18}F-fluorodeoxyglucose-positron emission tomography (^{18}F-FDG-PET) with computed tomography (CT) is a promising diagnostic tool for the diagnosis, evaluation, and the workup for vasculitis. Till recently, the accuracy and usefulness of ^{18}F-FDG-PET/CT as the diagnostic tool for vasculitis are debatable. However, PET-CT being the modality of choice for various pathologies, the localization of the incidental findings also leads to the specific interest resulting in more and more use of PET-CT in vasculitis. The use of PET-CT in the small cell vasculitis is not established with not many studies in favor of it.

© The Author(s), under exclusive license to Springer Nature
Singapore Pte Ltd. 2021
S. Shaikh, *PET-CT in Infection and Inflammation*,
https://doi.org/10.1007/978-981-15-9801-2_10

Vasculitis requires early diagnosis and initiation of treatment even if the diagnosis is uncertain. Vasculitis diagnosis is mostly based on the clinical symptoms and signs and correlating with the imaging findings. Usually, the diagnosis is done by the clinical examination, diagnostic workup of imaging, and laboratory findings. Vasculitis group usually shows raised inflammatory markers. Other markers of evaluation are the C-reactive protein, ESR, biopsies, and response to the steroid treatment. FDG PET-CT has an important role in the evaluation of large vessel vasculitis and medium vessel vasculitis [1–5].

FDG PET-CT in suspected cases is to be performed under whole-body protocol and if necessary upper and lower limbs to be scanned separately. A recommended protocol is CT angiogram followed by PET-CT. The concept of the angiogram is to delineate the vessel wall thickening and inflammation in the arterial phase as well as early changes of vasculitis which can be seen better, otherwise, in routine IV contrast study it will be venous phase where the vessel wall inflammation and enhancement cannot be ascertained.

^{18}F-FDG-PET/CT scan is considered positive when a linear uptake pattern is seen along the wall of the large arterial walls and/or its branches with an intensity similar or higher than the liver. A similar pattern of uptake is seen along the walls of the small- to medium-sized vasculitis is considered significant and may resemble the tree-root-like uptake pattern.

Arterial FDG uptake of lower density in suspected vessels can be diagnostic of primary large vessel vasculitis.

10.2   Vasculitis

Vasculitis is the inflammation of large- and medium-sized vessels. It is a clinico-pathological process with inflammation and destruction of the wall of the vessels. The vessel lumen is narrowed due to the ischemia of the tissue supplying the vessel wall. Different disease entities will be seen depending on the type, size, and location of a blood vessel may be involved. Usual involvement of vasculitis can be divided into small (Wegener's granulomatosis), medium (polyarteritis nodosa, Kawasaki's arteritis), and large vessel vasculitis (Takayasu's and giant-cell arteritis). Usually, it is an autoimmune disease caused by inflammation of large- and medium-sized vessels in the elderly age group of more than 50 years. Their deposition in vessel walls followed by neutrophil infiltration is the most common mechanism of vasculitic syndromes. As the process becomes subacute or chronic, this vasculitis may not be symptomatic and not diagnostic in diagnostic tests. Previously temporal artery biopsy was considered or specific and diagnostic tests for giant cell arteritis. However, temporal artery biopsy is moderately sensitive and has remarkably high false-negative rates from 15% to 66%. The giant cell arteritis is very crucial and needs urgent treatment. So, the diagnosis has to be very fast. Here PET-CT plays an important role in the early diagnostic workup of giant cell arteritis. This is in line with recent European league against rheumatism (EULAR) recommendations for the use of imaging in large cell vasculitis. This recommends early diagnosis by PET-CT.

^{18}F-FDG PET-CT the aorta and its main branches will show the normal background activity due to the less metabolically active cells dispersed between the many elastic layers of the arterial wall. In large-vessel vasculitis, the pattern of uptake will be abnormally representing as the linear pattern along the walls of the involved vessels, as shown in case reports of patients affected with systemic lupus erythematosus, Takayasu's arteritis, and giant cell arteritis (GCA). Giant cell arteritis is the primary cranial subtype affecting the extracranial arteries or primarily a large vessel subtype, which affects the aorta and its main branches [6–10]. The clinical symptoms of systemic inflammation such as fatigue, weight loss, fever, and night sweats, sometimes other findings such as limb claudication, large vessel bruits, pulselessness, and a combination of the above symptoms. Other nonspecific symptoms are headache, scalp tenderness, visual disturbances, and jaw claudication. This giant cell arteritis can also occur in combination with polymyalgia rheumatica [11]. Vessel wall inflammation reduces the amount of blood flow and can cause ischemic symptoms in form of vision loss, stroke, scalp, or tongue necrosis. The management of GCA is by early initiation of glucocorticoid therapy (steroid) (Figs. 10.1 and 10.2).

10.3   FDG PET-CT in Large Vessel Giant Cell Arteritis

Many studies have evaluated the role of FDG PET-CT and confirmed the inflammation in the aorta and its main branches. The first cohort study showed diagnostic accuracy with sensitivity of 92% and 71% and specificity of 85% and 91% with clinical diagnosis and biopsy as a reference [12–16]. In another study, FDG PET-CT showed significant diagnostic accuracy with meta-analysis revealing sensitivities of 80% to 90% and specificities of 89% to 98% using ACR criteria as a reference standard. One of the fallacies of FDG PET-CT is the reduced sensitivity due to immunosuppression and steroid therapy. This shows the significant role of FDG PET-CT ideally to be done before the therapy and after completion of therapy to have a precise comparison and evaluating the exact response of treatment [17] (Figs. 10.3 and 10.4).

10.4   Role of PET-CT in Cranial Giant Cell Arteritis

As per EULAR recommendations, FDG PET-CT is not diagnostic of cranial giant cell arteritis and is not recommended as first line of diagnosis. But with recent developments of modern PET-CT systems, the sensitivity has increased significantly. The sensitivity of cranial artery assessment has subsequently been reported in 75% of patients, which tap positive [18, 19].

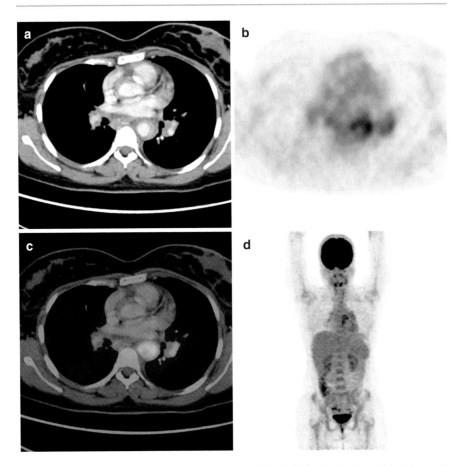

Fig. 10.1 CT showing diffuse irregular circumferential wall thickening in image (**a**) with associated mild metabolic activity SUV max of 3.5 along the ascending aorta, arch of aorta, descending thoracic aorta, and abdominal aorta in PET image (**b, d**) and fused image (**c**) suggestive of vasculitis

10.5 FDG PET-CT in Large Vessel Vasculitis

FDG PET-CT shows diffuse high FDG uptake along the walls of the large vessels consistent with vasculitis. Based on the available literature on expert consciences, the diagnostic criteria by FDG is FDG uptake in aorta and its main branches are graded according to liver FDG uptake (Grade-0: no vascular uptake, Grade-1: Vascular uptake < liver uptake, Grade-2: Vascular uptake = liver uptake, Grade-3: Vascular uptake > liver uptake) and Grade-3 is consistent with vasculitis while Grade-2 is diagnostic of vasculitis. This analysis is based on the uptake relative to the liver, which is quick without any measurements.

Large cell vasculitis usually involves the aorta, its main branches, and medium size extracranial arteries. Sometimes it can involve supra-aortic branches with or without infra-aortic arteries involvement [20–23] (Figs. 10.5 and 10.6).

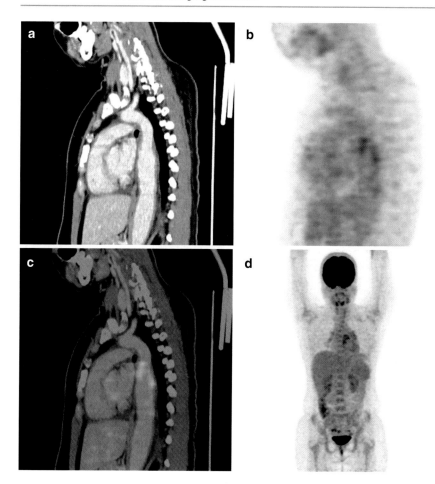

Fig. 10.2 CT showing diffuse irregular circumferential wall thickening in image (**a**) with associated mild metabolic activity SUV max of 3.5 along the ascending aorta, arch of aorta, descending thoracic aorta, and abdominal aorta in PET image (**b, d**) and fused image (**c**) suggestive of vasculitis

Various other conditions also cause large cell inflammation in conditions other than vasculitis like rheumatoid arthritis, Cogan syndrome, relapsing polychondritis, ankylosing spondylitis, systemic lupus erythematosus, Buerger's disease, Bechet's disease, inflammatory bowel disease, sarcoidosis, retroperitoneal fibrosis, immunoglobulin G4 disease, syphilis, and tuberculosis (Fig. 10.7).

10.6 FDG PET-CT Versus Other Imaging Modalities

FDG PET-CT has evolved as an important imaging technique that covers the entire body from the skull to thigh and upper and lower limbs as and when clinically indicated. FDG PET-CT showed the amount of tracer uptake along the vessel wall,

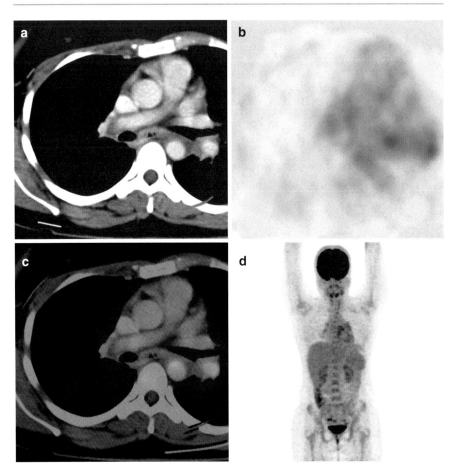

Fig. 10.3 CT showing diffuse irregular circumferential wall thickening in image (**a**) with associated mild metabolic activity SUV max of 3.5 along the ascending aorta, arch of aorta, descending thoracic aorta and abdominal aorta in PET image (**b**, **d**), and fused image (**c**) suggestive of vasculitis

which again depends on acute, chronic, or acute on chronic nature. The combination of PET-CT also defines the correct anatomical extent. Sometimes angiographic protocol is also done to define the exact nature of the wall, which can be missed in venous/delayed phase of angiogram. Thus, PET-CT is superior compared to other imaging modalities like CT, MR angiograms, which can define the extent of the wall, but the acute or chronic stage cannot be defined by these imaging modalities. This can be evaluated only by PET-CT.

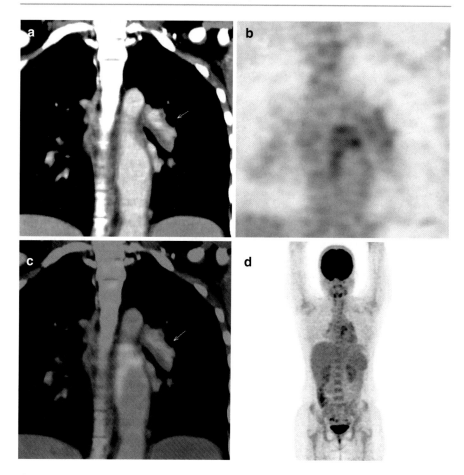

Fig. 10.4 CT showing diffuse irregular circumferential wall thickening in image (**a**) with associated mild metabolic activity SUV max of 3.5 along the ascending aorta, arch of aorta, descending thoracic aorta, and abdominal aorta in PET image (**b, d**) and fused image (**c**) suggestive of vasculitis

10.7   FDG PET in Monitoring Response to Therapy in Giant Cell Arteritis

Thus, the FDG PET-CT is important and acts as a biomarker of disease activity and also to evaluate the prognosis of the vasculitis depending on the extent of the disease, symptoms, and inflammation-associated treatments. Thus, FDG PET-CT is a valuable tool to monitor the treatment response in all other associated causes of vasculitis [24]. This makes it more important in the scenario of pre- and post-therapy evaluations (Fig. 10.8).

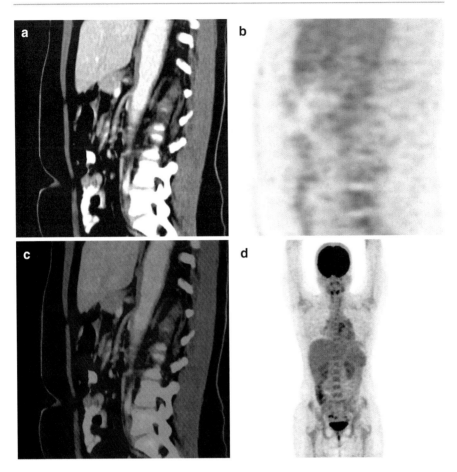

Fig. 10.5 PET-CT study, CT image (**a**) showing linear circumferential wall thickening with mild metabolic uptake involving descending thoracic aorta with SUV max of 3.5 in PET (**b**, **d**) and fused images (**c**) suggestive of large cell vasculitis

10.8   Vascular Graft Infection

Vascular graft infection is a rare complication of the graft with varying incidences from 0.5% to 5%. This may have very high mortality rate 25 to 88%. The diagnosis is not easy. The clinical presentation is non-specific and cannot redetect by conventional imaging modalities. FDG PET is important and having a great potential for the accuracy of this vascular graft infection. One of the studies by Fukuchi and colleagues [25] which showed superior sensitivity of FDG PET of 91% and specificity of 64% in comparison with CT sensitivity 64% and specificity 86%. If the uptake is focal and with positive criteria, both specificity and positive predictive values are increased by more than 95%. The amount of FDG uptake along the graft boundary,

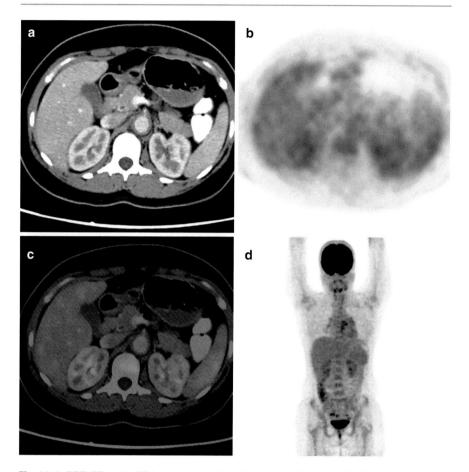

Fig. 10.6 PET-CT study, CT image (**a**) showing linear circumferential wall thickening with mild metabolic uptake involving descending thoracic aorta with SUV max of 3.5 in PET (**b**, **d**) and fused images (**c**) suggestive of large cell vasculitis

which can be focal or diffuse, mild, moderate, and intense, is a significant predictor of vascular graft infection. One of the major differences is diffuse uptake seen in the postoperative change, where true infection is associated with focal FDG uptake. FDG PET has also been shown to be valuable for the assessment of vascular graft infection.

10.9 Takayasu's Disease

The evaluation of Takayasu's disease is based on the same findings of the other large cell vasculitis by diffuse or focal uptake which is noted depending on the amount of infection and inflammation in the medium vessels [26]. Same principle of pre and post therapy evaluation also applies here for monitering response to theraphy.

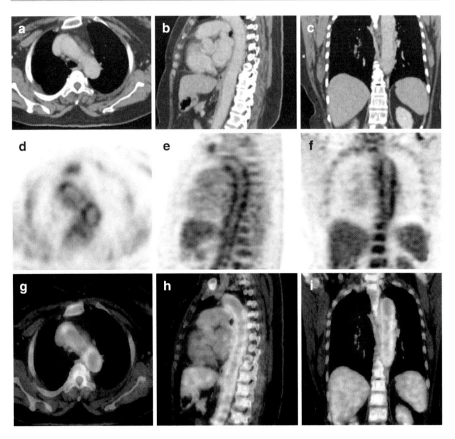

Fig. 10.7 Whole-body PET-CT with chest images showing circumferential wall thickening on CT image (**a–c**) with corresponding diffuse metabolic uptake seen in fused (**g–i**)and PET images (**d–f**) with SUV max of 4.2 suggestive of active vasculitis

10.10 PET-MRI

With the advent of PET-MRI, the characteristic finding and evaluation have become more sensitive and specific. There are three patterns of inflammation defined on abnormal PET and MRI findings. PET-MRI is having the capability of quantitative radiotracer uptake along with multi-contrast anatomic assessment of MRI along with PET in one scan. The two entities are defined by imaging characteristics of the inflammatory pattern which suggests the presence of inflammatory process where is fibrous pattern suggest fibrotic lesions. Compared with PET-CT, PET-MRI has the biggest advantage of no radiation to the patient and can be used repeatedly to determine the remission, progression, or absence of the lesion. Another advantage is the use of gadolinium or the wall enhancement. PET-MRI can be an excellent

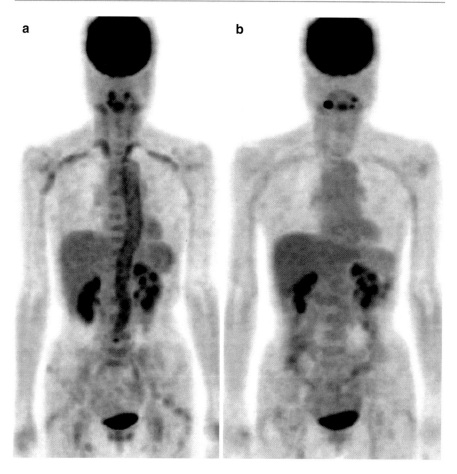

Fig. 10.8 PET image (**a**) showing pre-therapy status of vasculitis involving thoracic and abdominal aorta. PET image (**b**) showing complete resolution of linear uptake after glucocorticoid therapy suggestive of complete remission

alternative with significant functional imaging capabilities and can easily characterize the disease activity in the challenging cases [27].

10.11   Conclusion

Thus, FDG PET-CT has high diagnostic accuracy and must be evaluated to define the intensity, pattern, and distribution based on the clinical condition and to differentiate from other differential diagnosis. With this advancement in PET-CT, the sensitivity and specificity of vasculitis evaluation will become more precise and accurate.

References

1. Bleeker-Rovers CP, Bredie SJ, van der Meer JW, Corstens FH, Oyen WJ. 18F-fluorodeoxyglucose positron emission tomography in diagnosis and follow-up of patients with different types of vasculitis. Neth J Med. 2003;61:323–9.
2. Prieto-Gonzalez S, Arguis P, Cid MC. Imaging in systemic vasculitis. Curr Opin Rheumatol. 2015;27(1):53–62.
3. Soussan M, Nicolas P, Schramm C, et al. Management of large-vessel vasculitis with FDG-PET. Medicine. 2015;94(14):e622.
4. Weyand CM, Goronzy JJ. Giant-cell arteritis and polymyalgia rheumatica. N Engl J Med. 2014;371(17):1652–3.
5. Prieto-Gonzalez S, Depetris M, Garcia-Martinez A, et al. Positron emission tomography assessment of large vessel inflammation in patients with newly diagnosed, biopsy proven giant cell arteritis: a prospective, case-control study. Ann Rheum Dis. 2014;73(7):1388–92.
6. Fuchs M, Briel M, Daikeler T, et al. The impact of 18F-FDG PET on the management of patients with suspected large vessel vasculitis. Eur J Nucl Med Mol Imaging. 2012;39(2):344–53.
7. Soussan M, Abisror N, Abad S, et al. FDG-PET/CT in patients with ANCA-associated vasculitis: case-series and literature review. Autoimmun Rev. 2014;13(2):125–31.
8. Kemna MJ, Vandergheynst F, Vöö S, et al. Positron emission tomography scanning in anti-neutrophil cytoplasmic antibodies-associated vasculitis. Medicine. 2015;94(20):e747.
9. Nielsen BD, Gormsen LC, Hansen IT, Keller KK, Therkildsen P, Hauge E-M. Three days of high-dose glucocorticoid treatment attenuates large-vessel 18F-FDG uptake in large-vessel giant cell arteritis but with a limited impact on diagnostic accuracy. Eur J Nucl Med Mol Imaging. 2018;45(7):1119–28.
10. Blockmans D, De Ceuninck L, Vanderschueren S, Knockaert D, Mortelmans L, Bobbaers H. Repetitive 18F-fluorodeoxyglucose positron emission tomography in giant cell arteritis: a prospective study of 35 patients. Arthritis Rheum. 2006;55(1):131–7.
11. Buttgereit F, Dejaco C, Matteson EL, Dasgupta B. Polymyalgia rheumatica and giant cell arteritis. JAMA. 2016;315(22):2442.
12. Clifford AH, Murphy EM, Burrell SC, et al. Positron emission tomography/computerized tomography in newly diagnosed patients with giant cell arteritis who are taking glucocorticoids. J Rheumatol. 2017;44(12):1859–66.
13. Imfeld S, Rottenburger C, Schegk E, et al. [18F]FDG positron emission tomography in patients presenting with suspicion of giant cell arteritis—lessons from a vasculitis clinic. Eur Heart J Cardiovasc Imaging. 2017;19(8):933–40.
14. Besson FL, Parienti J-J, Bienvenu B, et al. Diagnostic performance of 18F-fluorodeoxyglucose positron emission tomography in giant cell arteritis: a systematic review and meta-analysis. Eur J Nucl Med Mol Imaging. 2011;38(9):1764–72.
15. Puppo C, Massollo M, Paparo F, et al. Giant cell arteritis: a systematic review of the qualitative and semiquantitative methods to assess vasculitis with 18F-fluorodeoxyglucose positron emission tomography. In: BioMed Res Int; 2014. https://doi.org/10.1155/2014/574248.
16. Einspieler I, Thurmel K, Eiber M. Fully integrated whole-body [18F]-fludeoxyglucose positron emission tomography/magnetic resonance imaging in therapy monitoring of giant cell arteritis. Eur Heart J. 2016;37:576. https://doi.org/10.1093/eurheartj/ehv607.
17. Prieto-Gonzalez S, Garcia-Martinez A, Tavera-Bahillo I, Hernandez-Rodriguez J, Gutierrez-Chacoff J, Alba MA, et al. Effect of glucocorticoid treatment on computed tomography angiography detected large-vessel inflammation in giant-cell arteritis. A prospective, longitudinal study. Medicine (Baltimore). 2015;94:e486. https://doi.org/10.1097/MD.0000000000000486.
18. Dejaco C, Ramiro S, Duftner C, et al. EULAR recommendations for the use of imaging in large vessel vasculitis in clinical practice. Ann Rheumatic Dis. 2018;77(5):636–43.
19. Slart RHJA, Writing Group, Reviewer Group, et al. FDGPET/CT(A) imaging in large vessel vasculitis and polymyalgia rheumatica: joint procedural recommendation of the EANM,

SNMMI, and the PET interest group (PIG), and endorsed by the ASNC. Eur J Nucl Med Mol Imaging. 2018;45(7):1250–69.

20. Muto G, Yamashita H, Takahashi Y, Miyata Y, Morooka M, Minamimoto R, et al. Large vessel vasculitis in elderly patients: early diagnosis and steroid-response evaluation with FDG-PET/CT and contrast-enhanced CT. Rheumatol Int. 2014;34:1545–54. https://doi.org/10.1007/s00296-014-2985-3.

21. Martínez-Rodríguez I, Jimenez-Alonso M, Quirce R, et al. 18F-FDG PET/CT in the follow-up of large-vessel vasculitis: a study of 37 consecutive patients. Semin Arthritis Rheum. 2018;47(4):530–7.

22. Papathanasiou ND, Du Y, Menezes LJ, et al. 18F-fludeoxyglucose PET/CT in the evaluation of large-vessel vasculitis: diagnostic performance and correlation with clinical and laboratory parameters. Br J Radiol. 2012;85(1014):e188–94.

23. Bertagna F, Bosio G, Caobelli F, Motta F, Biasiotto G, Giubbini R. Role of 18F-fluorodeoxyglucose positron emission tomography/computed tomography for therapy evaluation of patients with large-vessel vasculitis. Jpn J Radiol. 2010;28:199–204. https://doi.org/10.1007/s11604-009-0408-2.

24. Langford CA, Cuthbertson D, Ytterberg SR, Khalidi N, Monach PA, Carette S, et al. A randomized, double-blind trial of Abatacept (CTLA-4Ig) for the treatment of Takayasu arteritis. Arthritis Rheumatol. 2017;69:846–53. https://doi.org/10.1002/art.40037.

25. Fukuchi K, Ishida Y, Higashi M, et al. Detection of aortic graft infection by fluorodeoxyglucose positron emission tomography: comparison with computed tomographic findings. J Vasc Surg. 2005;42:919–25.

26. Johnston SL, Lock RJ, Gompels MM. Takayasu arteritis: a review. J Clin Pathol. 2002;55:481–6.

27. Einspieler I, et al. Imaging large vessel vasculitis with fully integrated PET/MRI: a pilot study. Eur J Nucl Med Mol Imaging. 2015;42:1012–24.

PET-CT in Tuberculosis

11

Key Points

Tuberculosis is one of the most common infections worldwide, which has very high morbidity and mortality. Tuberculosis is caused by *Mycobacterium tuberculosis* and having a complex pathology. It is the aerobic bacillus capable of surviving in anaerobic conditions. It can be diagnosed based on the epidemiology, symptoms, and additional tests and specific and nonspecific signs and symptoms. However, in the Indian subcontinent, it is still the commonest form of infection. It is caused by *Mycobacterium tuberculosis* (MTB) which is an aerobic bacillus that survives in anaerobic conditions for a very long time. PET-CT has become an important imaging modality for diagnosis staging and assessing therapy response.

11.1 Introduction

Molecular imaging is based on PET-CT, which can provide a three-dimensional view of the disease in the entire body at a time. The role of PET-CT is now commonly used to differentiate between tuberculosis and malignant concurrent conditions at same time.

Tuberculosis remains the biggest threat to humans, especially due to various causes, multidrug resistance, and immune-compromised status are one of the commonest. TB has one of the highest mortalities [1–3]. The commonest reason for the increased morbidity and mortality is multidrug-resistant TB (MDRTB) and immune-compromised status [4].

© The Author(s), under exclusive license to Springer Nature
Singapore Pte Ltd. 2021
S. Shaikh, *PET-CT in Infection and Inflammation*,
https://doi.org/10.1007/978-981-15-9801-2_11

11.2   Pathophysiology

Mycobacterium tuberculi is an aerobic intracellular microorganism with thick cell walls having long chain of fatty acids called mycolic acids. This MTB has the peculiarity to persist in the host cells dormant for a long time [5]. The commonest mode of spread of this is through droplets as aerosol generated through the respiratory system. The risk of development of pulmonary tuberculosis is based on endogenous and exogenous factors. Exogenous factors will have a role from exposure to infection while endogenous factors have a role from infection to active disease. Again, it depends on the PTB and extra PTB were a lot of factors are influencing. The activation of the immune system cells boosts the cell glycolysis even in the scenario of the immune suppression. With this, there will be increased glycolysis resulting in the increased FDG uptake. MTB can be defined clinically by tuberculin skin test, which is still not sensitive. The characteristic feature of MTB is slow growth and dormant, latent persistent state. MTB is transmitted by aerosol generated by the respiratory tract and is primary source of infection, which is labeled as primary tuberculosis. The commonest location for primary tuberculosis is the lung, which has varied features imaging wise and shows different phases depending on the treatment.

11.3   Clinical Symptoms

The classical clinical features are chronic cough, weight loss, fever, night sweats, and hemoptysis. The predisposing factors are mal-rotation, tobacco smoking, and pollution. The extrapulmonary TB occurs in 10% to 42% and depends on the age presence or absence of underlying disease, human status of an individual, and strain of MTB. Diagnosis of tuberculosis is done by Mantoux tuberculin skin test. Imaging in a tuberculosis chest radiograph is the most commonly used diagnostic imaging modality for pulmonary tuberculosis. Varied presentations are seen depending on the various factors. This can be patchy opacities, cavitation's, fibrosis, nodal involvement, and with or without caseation necrosis. Conventional radiograph is also used in other extrapulmonary tuberculosis, which is not highly sensitive [6]. For these other modalities like ultrasound, CT, and MRI are used depending on the organ or systemic involvement.

11.4   PET-CT

PET-CT is a combination of molecular and anatomical information with this it has an ability to evaluate the various aspects of the disease [7, 8]. FDG PET-CT is to evaluate the anatomical, microbiological, immunologic, and pharmacological components related to tuberculosis. FDG PET-CT is nonspecific for the evaluation as many malignant pathologies and inflammatory conditions which has an overlap of many conditions, they also demonstrate similar uptake patterns. Tuberculosis is classified into two major groups: Pulmonary tuberculosis and Non-Pulmonary tuberculosis. The role of PET-CT now is well established and documented to detect the tuberculosis disease activity [9–13] and extent of disease. The capacity of FDG PET to distinguish between benign and malignant lesions is being evolved with encouraging results. FDG PET shows diffuse increased uptake in both pulmonary and extrapulmonary lesions and helps to assess the extent of the active disease. PET has an advantage though not sensitive to distinguish between malignancy and other granulomatous conditions. Thus, there is a significant overlap between the SUV values in malignant, benign, and other granulomatous lesions, but recent studies that show the dual time point imaging which is a delayed PET imaging to distinguish between benign and malignant lesions. The concept theory is after doing dual point imaging, the SUV values will be falling in cases of infective inflammatory, tuberculosis, and granulomatous pathologies. However, malignant tissues will have a capacity to retain the radiotracer, which is the characteristic feature of the malignant pathology [14]. Now tuberculosis involving the cerebral parenchyma known as tuberculomas or sometimes difficult to differentiate between malignant gliomas, fungal infections, and other granulomas. FDG uptake can be quantified to evaluate the intracerebral lesions and meningeal and Dural involvement in phases like tuberculous meningitis or tubercular meningoencephalitis [15]. Diffuse uptake will be noted in the lesion along the meninges or the dura. Same applies to the spinal cord that can be involving the spinal cord parenchyma and the arachnoid space.

Other radiotracers like 11C Choline, 68 Ga-Citrate, and 18 F FLT are in pipeline and will be used in coming years.

Another set of newer radiotracers that are in the preclinical stage are 11C Rifampicin, 11C Pyrazinamide, 11C Isoniazid, and 18F NaF and these radiotracers will be more specific and precise for the evaluation of MDRT or extrapulmonary tuberculosis. Hypoxia PET imaging will also be a promising radiotracer in the future.

11.5 Head and Neck Tuberculosis

Intracranial tuberculosis is one of the common pathologies, which shows features similar to neoplastic lesions. Ring enhancing lesion with perilesional edema is one of the common features. These lesions show increased metabolic activity (Figs. 11.1 and 11.2).

The commonest tubercular involvement in the neck is in form of lymph nodes. The presentation of nodal involvement depends on the stage of the disease activity within the node [16]. Again the SUV value varies according to the stage and phase of tuberculosis. In suspected cases, dual point imaging can be used to distinguish between tuberculosis vs. malignant pathologies (Fig. 11.3).

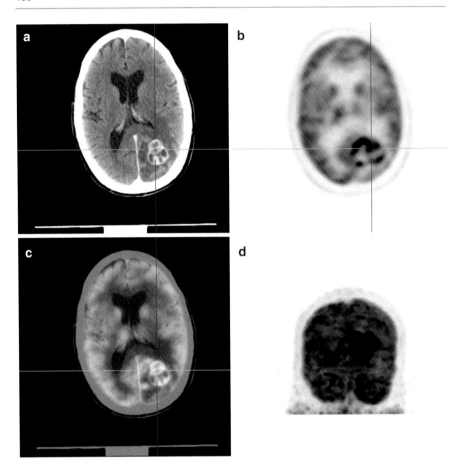

Fig. 11.1 Brain PET-CT, CT image (**a**) showing lobulated ring-enhancing lesion with irregular soft tissue component in the left parieto-occipital region increased metabolic activity in PET images (**b, d**) and fused image (**c**) with SUV max of 5.8 suggestive of tuberculoma

11.6   Chest

The commonest tuberculosis presentation is pulmonary tuberculosis. Varied presentations in the form of patchy infiltrates, nodules, consolidations, collapse, focal pleural thickening, cavitation's, ectatic changes, ground glass opacities, honeycombing, pleural effusion, mediastinal nodes, and combination of the above-mentioned entities. The presentation of especially mediastinal nodes depends on the phase of the disease, active disease, caseation necrosis, or calcifications. Tuberculosis involving the chest wall muscles is also equally common in the Indian subcontinent. Tuberculosis involving the pericardium is quite common and presents clinically in the form of pericarditis and severe cases of pericardial tamponade [17]. It can be focal pleural involvement or diffuse pleural involvement with or without pericardial

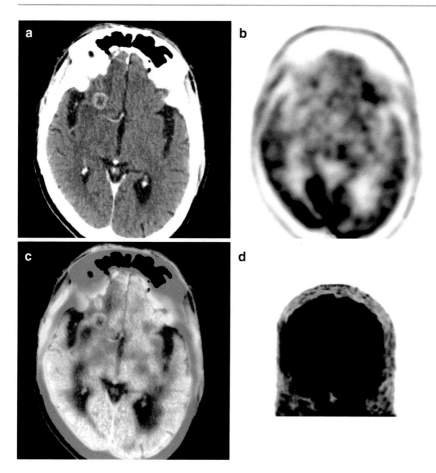

Fig. 11.2 Small ring-enhancing lesion on CT image (**a**) with mild peripheral uptake on PET and fused images (**b, d, c**) with SUV max of 2.5. This was later diagnosed as tuberculoma

effusion. In chronic cases, there will be calcification of the pericardium representing as constrictive pericarditis. The role of PET-CT is to evaluate the active disease and to differentiate between other neoplastic differentials [18, 19] (Figs. 11.4, 11.5, 11.6, and 11.7).

11.7 Abdomen

Tuberculosis involving the abdomen is mostly confined to GI tract and GUT. GIT stomach is very rarely involved [20]. Small intestine is not common except ileocecal junction, which is very commonest cause of GI tuberculosis. Colon is not commonly involved by tuberculosis. The ileocecal Koch's is the commonest form of tuberculosis with close differential with Crohn's disease, ulcerative colitis, and

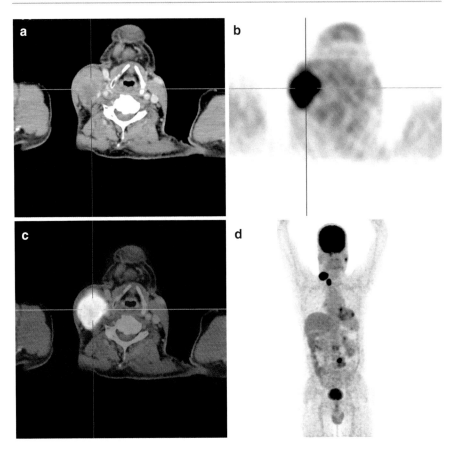

Fig. 11.3 Enlarged patchily enhancing lymph nodes in CT image (**a**) in right level-III and IV with significantly increased uptake on PET images (**b**, **d**) and fused image (**c**) with SUV max of 9 suggestive of necrotic caseating tuberculous nodes

ileocecal malignancies [21]. PET-CT has an important role in quantification of the SUV values. Again, dual point imaging is based on important role in differentiating between Koch's and malignant pathologies.

11.8   Genito Urinary Tract

Renal tuberculosis is also an important and common cause with varied presentations. The presentations involving the focal or diffuse renal involvement that can be acute or chronic depending on the stage and time of the disease [22, 23]. Renal pelvicalyceal system is also involved with varied presentations. Tuberculosis involvement of ureter is not common, but literature and PET-CT shows diffuse increased uptake involving the ureter, which can be focal, diffuse stricture, or hydronephrosis [24]. One of the commonest forms of tuberculosis is involving the

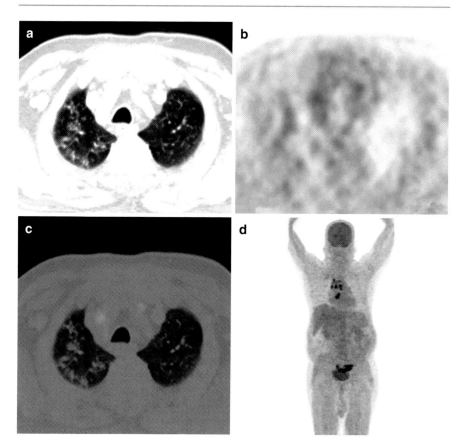

Fig. 11.4 Whole-body PET-CT, CT image (**a**) showing patchy parenchymal infiltrates with mild metabolic activity in the right upper lobe in PET (**b, d**) and fused images (**c**), respectively, with SUV max of 3.4. Small metabolically active mediastinal nodes. Findings are suggestive of pulmonary tuberculosis

urinary bladder. It can be focal or diffuse with perivesical involvement. Tuberculosis involving prostate which can be focal or diffuse. Small nodule, abscess, or may present as prostatitis. PET has an important role to differentiate between nodular lesions that can be tubercular or malignant [25, 26]. FDG PET-CT has extremely low sensitivity for prostatic malignancies [27]. The newer radiotracer Prostate-Specific Membrane Antigen (PSMA) is being widely used for prostatic malignancies and has remarkably high sensitivity compared to FDG PET [28]. This is very sensitive for infective inflammatory and tubercular lesions, which can be quantified by SUV max values. Tuberculosis of the urethra is an important entity in the Indian subcontinent. The commonest presentation is in the form of stricture and urethritis. PET-CT plays an important role in the quantification of tuberculosis pathology (Fig. 11.8).

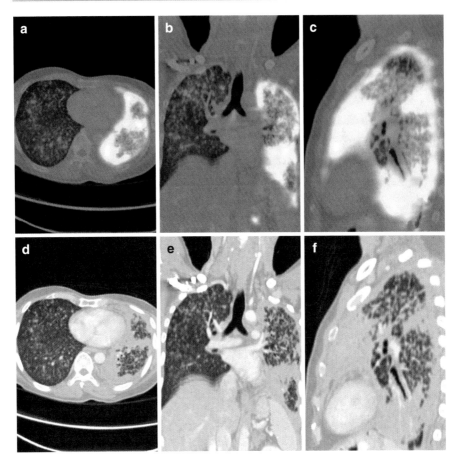

Fig. 11.5 Whole-body PET-CT showing a significant loss of left lung volume with diffuse nodular pleural thickening on left side with significant metabolic activity in PET-CT fused images (**a–c**) with SUV max of 7.8. Diffuse miliary mottling noted in both lungs also seen in both lungs in CT images (**d–f**)

11.9   Female Pelvis

Female genitourinary tuberculosis is the commonest cause involving non-oncological pathologies that can be in the form of salpingo-oophoritis, which is the commonest cause of tuberculosis. PET-CT shows diffuse increased uptake in the organs of involvement and in the post ATT evaluation. Uterine tuberculosis is not that much common but endometrial involvement is the commonest form. PET-CT plays an important role in differentiating endometrial malignancy, endometritis, endometriosis, and endometrial tuberculosis [24, 29].

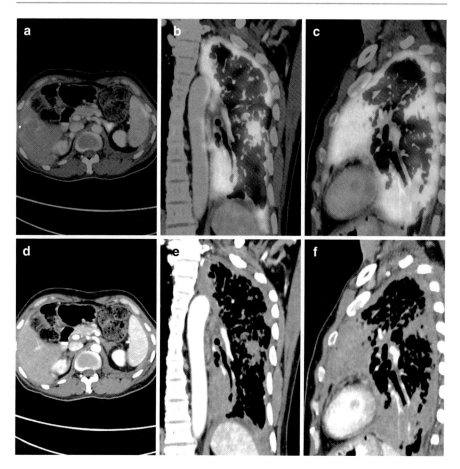

Fig. 11.6 Whole-body PET-CT showing a significant loss of left lung volume with diffuse nodular pleural thickening on left side with significant metabolic activity in PET-CT fused images (**a–c**) with SUV max of 7.8. Diffuse miliary mottling noted in both lungs also seen in both lungs in CT images (**d–f**)

11.10 Peritoneum

Peritoneal tuberculosis is one of the important commonest causes of abdominal tuberculosis. It can be focal or diffuse nodular or mass lesions with or without ascites. The PET-CT plays an important role in differentiating between pseudomyxoma peritonei (which is a primary peritoneal tumor) vs. peritoneal tuberculosis [30] (Fig. 11.9).

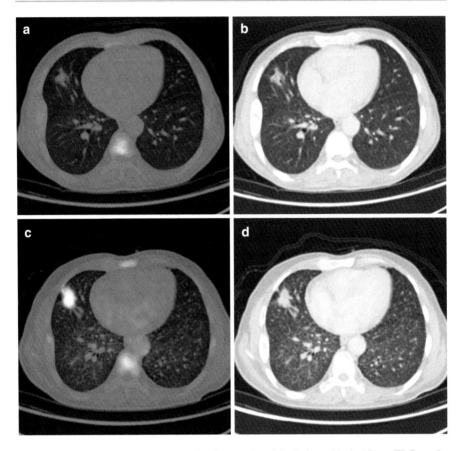

Fig. 11.7 PET-CT at the level of chest showing small nodular lesion with significant FDG uptake in right upper lobe with SUV max of 5.8 in PET-CT fused images (**a, c**). Associated miliary mottling in both lower lobes seen in the CT images (**b, d**). Findings are suggestive of pulmonary Koch's

11.11 Musculoskeletal

Musculoskeletal tuberculosis is one of the important extrapulmonary forms of tuberculosis. It can involve the axial or appendicular skeleton.

11.11.1 Axial Skeleton

Axial skeleton which can be seen in the form of tubercular discitis, psoas abscess, vertebral body involvement, prevertebral, paravertebral, and epidural soft tissue component with abscess formations depending on the stage of the disease. Vertebral

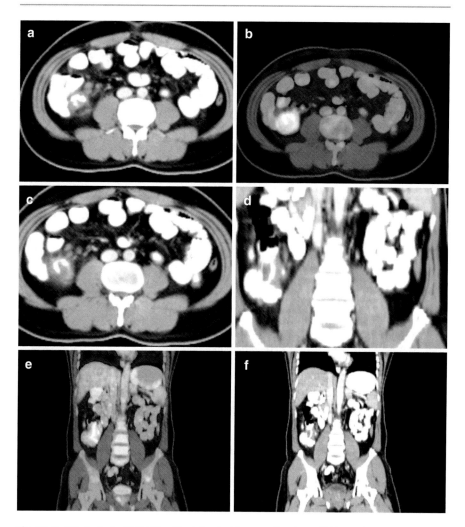

Fig. 11.8 Whole-body PET-CT with abdominal images showing mild irregular wall thickening involving the ileocecal junction and adjacent small nodes in CT images (**a, c, d**, and **f**). This wall thickening shows increased uptake with SUV max of 6.9 in fused images (**b, e**) suggestive of ileo-cecal tuberculosis

involvement may lead to destruction of the vertebral bodies, collapse compression fractures and spinal cord involvement, and cervical and dorsal regions. There can be associated involvement of the spinal canal and spinal cord. FDG PET-CT is an excellent modality to evaluate the tuberculosis involving axial skeleton. One of the commonest forms is lumbar vertebral tuberculosis with psoas abscess [31] (Fig. 11.10).

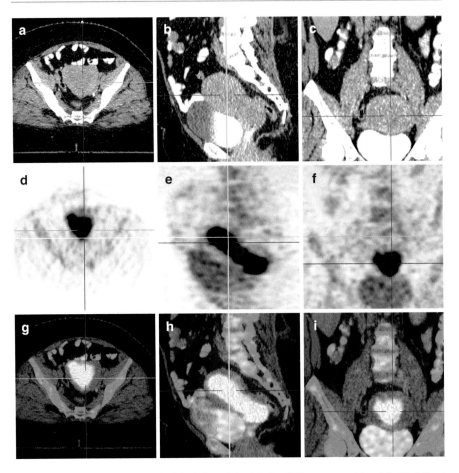

Fig. 11.9 Limited abdomen PET-CT of the pelvis showing bulky uterus with subtle ill-defined hypodense soft tissue in the endometrial cavity on CT images (**a–c**). PET (**d–f**) and fused images (**g–i**) show diffuse extensive metabolic activity corresponding to the hypodense lesion in the endometrium with SUV max of 11.8. Histopathologically suggestive of endometrial tuberculosis

11.11.2   Appendicular Skeleton

11.11.2.1   Hip Joint

The commonest form of tuberculosis are joint involvement, synovial thickening, joint effusion, bony erosions, bony destructions, and associated features like soft tissue and neural involvement. PET-CT has an important role in quantifying the amount of uptake by SUV values [32].

11.11.2.2   Knee Joint, Shoulder Joint, Ankle Joint, and Elbow Joint

The commonest form of tuberculosis joint involvement, synovial thickening, joint effusion, bony erosions, bony destructions, and associated features like deformities.

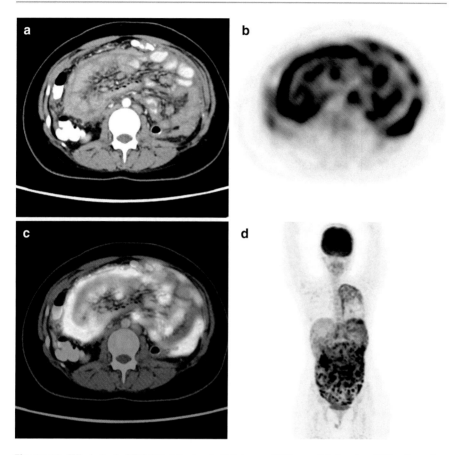

Fig. 11.10 Whole-body PET-CT at the level of abdomen CT image (**a**) showing diffuse irregular peritoneal thickening with cocoon formation with metabolic uptake in PET images (**b**, **d**) and fused image (**c**) showing SUV max of 7.7. Findings are suggestive of peritoneal tuberculosis

A small joint tuberculosis are rarely involved. PET-CT has an important role to differentiating between the associated pathologies involving the joints [33–37].

11.11.3   Muscles

The commonest presentation of tuberculosis involving the muscle is the psoas abscess. Other features presenting the muscles are focal bulkiness and small collections or abscess involving the muscles. The PET has an important role in quantifying the SUV values [38]. However, clinical correlation is important to differentiate between infective inflammatory and tubercular pathologies (Fig. 11.11).

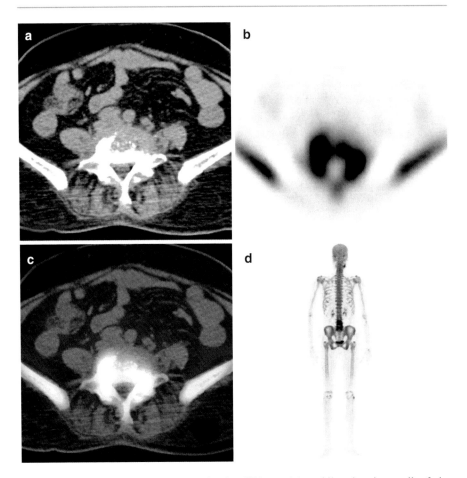

Fig. 11.11 Whole-body F-18 bone scan showing CT image (**a**) patchily enhancing small soft tissue component in the prevertebral and bilateral paravertebral locations with significant uptake in fused (**c**) and PET images (**b, d**) at L4–L5 level suggestive of Pott's spine

11.12 Conclusion

PET-CT is a sensitive biomarker for detection, staging, accessing the disease activity, and monitoring response to therapy since tuberculosis has long treatment regimes. PET-CT offers the early option for the posttreatment evaluation, especially in relation to the short regimes as the drugs can be modified if needed thus reducing the morbidity and mortality. With the advent of MDRT and newer radiotracers, the role of PET-CT is more consolidated in the future.

References

1. Ankrah AO, Glaudemans AWJM, Maes A, et al. Tuberculosis. Semin Nucl Med. 2018;48(2):108–30.
2. Burrill J, Williams CJ, Bain G, et al. Tuberculosis: a radiologic review. Radiographics. 2007;27(5):1255–73.
3. Gambhir S, Ravina M, Rangan K, et al. Imaging in extra-pulmonary tuberculosis. Int J Infect Dis. 2017;56:237–47.
4. Choi J, Jhun B, Hyun S, et al. 18F-Fluorodeoxyglucose positron emission tomography/computed tomography for assessing treatment response of pulmonary multidrug-resistant tuberculosis. J Clin Med. 2018;7(12):559.
5. Patrick Cudahy MD, Sheela Shenoi MD. Diagnostics for pulmonary tuberculosis. Postgrad Med J. 2016 Apr;92(1086):187–93.
6. Martin C, Castaigne C, Vierasu I, et al. Prospective serial FDG PET/CT during treatment of extra-pulmonary tuberculosis in HIV-infected patients: an exploratory study. Clin Nucl Med. 2018;43(9):635–40.
7. Sathekge M, Maes A, CVD W. FDG-PET imaging in HIV infection and tuberculosis. Semin Nucl Med. 2013;43(5):349–66.
8. Geadas C, Acuna-Villaorduna C, Mercier G, et al. FDG-PET/CT activity leads to the diagnosis of unsuspected TB: a retrospective study. BMC Res Notes. 2018;11(1):464.
9. Vorster M, Sathekge MM, Bomanji J. Advances in imaging of tuberculosis: the role of 18F-FDG PET and PET/CT. Curr Opin Pulm Med. 2014;20(3):287–93.
10. Martinez V, Castilla-Lievre MA, Guillet-Caruba C, et al. ^{18}F-FDG PET/CT in tuberculosis: an early non-invasive marker of therapeutic response. Int J Tuberc Lung Dis. 2012;16(9):1180–5.
11. Ito K, Morooka M, Minamimoto R, et al. Imaging spectrum and pitfalls of ^{18}F-fluorodeoxyglucose positron emission tomography/computed tomography in patients with tuberculosis. Jpn J Radiol. 2013;31(8):511–20.
12. Agarwal KK, Behera A, Kumar R, et al. ^{18}F-Fluoro-deoxyglucose positron emission tomography/computed tomography in tuberculosis: spectrum of manifestations. Indian J Nucl Med. 2017;32(4):316–21.
13. Yu H-Y, Sheng J-F. Liver tuberculosis presenting as an uncommon cause of pyrexia of unknown origin: positron emission tomography/computed tomography identifies the correct site for biopsy. Med Princ Pract. 2014;23(6):577–9.
14. Maturu VN, Agarwal R, Aggarwal AN, et al. Dual-time point whole-body 18F-fluorodeoxyglucose PET/CT imaging in undiagnosed mediastinal lymphadenopathy: a prospective study of 117 patients with sarcoidosis and TB. Chest. 2014;146(6):e216–20.
15. Gambhir S, Kumar M, Ravina M, et al. Role of 18F-FDG PET in demonstrating disease burden in patients with tuberculous meningitis. J Neurol Sci. 2016;370:196–200.
16. Lefebvre N, Argemi X, Meyer N, et al. Clinical usefulness of 18F-FDG PET/CT for initial staging and assessment of treatment efficacy in patients with lymphnode tuberculosis. Nucl Med Biol. 2017;50:17–24.
17. Testempassi E, Kubota K, Morooka M, et al. Constrictive tuberculous pericarditis diagnosed using 18 F-fluorodeoxyglucose positron emission tomography: a report of two cases. Ann Nucl Med. 2010;24(5):421–5.
18. Li Y, Su M, Li F, et al. The value of ^{18}F-FDG-PET/CT in the differential diagnosis of solitary pulmonary nodules in areas with a high incidence of tuberculosis. Ann Nucl Med. 2011;25(10):804–11.
19. Demura Y, Tsuchida T, Uesaka D, et al. Usefulness of 18 F-fluorodeoxyglucose positron emission tomography for diagnosing disease activity and monitoring therapeutic response in patients with pulmonary mycobacteriosis. Eur J Nucl Med Mol Imaging. 2009;36(4):632–9.
20. Akdogan RA, Rakici H, Gungor S, et al. F-18 Fluoro-deoxyglucose positron emission tomography/computed tomography findings of isolated gastric tuberculosis mimicking gastric cancer and lymphoma. Euroasian J Hepatogastroenterol. 2018;8(1):93.

21. Ankrah AO, van der Werf TS, de Vries EFJ, Dierckx RAJO, Sathekge MM, Glaudemans AWJM. PET/CT imaging of *Mycobacterium tuberculosis* infection. Clin Transl Imaging. 2016;4:131–44.
22. Zhuang H, Pourdehnad M, Lambright ES, Yamamoto AJ, Lanuti M, Li P, Mozley PD, Rossman MD, Albelda SM, Alavi A. Dual time point ^{18}F-FDG PET imaging for differentiating malignant from inflammatory processes. J Nucl Med. 2001;42:1412–7.
23. Kubota K, Itoh M, Ozaki K, Ono S, Tashiro M, Yamaguchi K, Akaizawa T, Yamada K, Fukuda H. Advantage of delayed whole-body FDG-PET imaging for tumour detection. Eur J Nucl Med. 2001;28:696–703.
24. Sharma JB, Karmakar D, Kumar R, Shamim SA, Kumar S, Singh N, et al. Comparison of PET/CT with other imaging modalities in women with genital tuberculosis. Int J Gynaecol Obstet. 2012;118:123–8.
25. da Rocha EL, Pedrassa BC, Bormann RL, Kierszenbaum ML, Torres LR, D'Ippolito G. Abdominal tuberculosis: a radiological review with emphasis on computed tomography and magnetic resonance imaging findings. Radiol Bras. 2015;48:181–91.
26. Muneer A, Macrae B, Krishnamoorthy S, Zumla A. Urogenital tuberculosis - epidemiology, pathogenesis and clinical features. Nat Rev Urol. 2019 Oct;16(10):573–98.
27. Kulchavenya E, Kim CS, Bulanova O, Zhukova I. Male genital tuberculosis: epidemiology and diagnostic. World J Urol. 2012;30:15–21.
28. Koerber SA, Utzinger MT, Kratochwil C, et al. ^{68}Ga-PSMA11-PET/CT in newly diagnosed carcinoma of the prostate: correlation of intraprostatic PSMA uptake with several clinical parameters. J Nucl Med. 2017;58(12):1943–8.
29. Merchant S, Bharati A, Merchant N. Tuberculosis of the genitourinary system-urinary tract tuberculosis: renal tuberculosis-part II. Indian J Radiol Imaging. 2013;23:64–77.
30. Chen R, Chen Y, Liu L, et al. The role of 18F-FDG PET/CT in the evaluation of peritoneal thickening of undetermined origin. Medicine. 2016;95(15):e3023.
31. Kilborn T, Janse van Rensburg P, Candy S. Pediatric and adult spinal tuberculosis: imaging and pathophysiology. Neuroimaging Clin N Am. 2015;25:209–31.
32. Makis W, Abikhzer G, et al. Tuberculous synovitis of the hip joint diagnosed by FDGPET-CT. Clin Nucl Med. July 2009;34(7):431–2.
33. Wang J-H, Chi C-Y, Lin K-H, Ho M-W. Tuberculous arthritis—unexpected extra-pulmonary tuberculosis detected by FDG PET/CT. Clin Nucl Med. 2013 Feb;38(2):e93–4.
34. Ostrowska M, Gietka J, Nesteruk T, et al. Shoulder joint tuberculosis. Pol J Radiol. 2012 Oct–Dec;77(4):55–9.
35. Grayson PC, Alehashemi S, Bagheri AA, Civelek AC, Cupps TR, Kaplan MJ, et al. ^{18}F-Fluorodeoxyglucose-positron emission tomography as an imaging biomarker in a prospective, longitudinal cohort of patients with large vessel vasculitis. Arthritis Rheumatol. 2018;70(3):439–49.
36. Selçuk NA, Fenercioğlu A, Selçuk HH, et al. Multifoci bone tuberculosis and lymphadenitis in mediastinum mimics malignancy on FDG-PET/CT: a case report. Mol Imaging Radionucl Ther. 2014 Feb;23(1):39–42.
37. Singhal S, Arbart A, Lanjewar A, Ranjan R. Tuberculous dactylitis—a rare manifestation of adult skeletal tuberculosis. Indian J Tuberc. 2005;52:218–9.
38. Kang K, Lim I, Roh JK. Positron emission tomographic findings in a tuberculous abscess. Ann Nucl Med. 2007;21:303–6.

PET-CT in Immunocompromised Status

12

Key Points

Immunocompromised status is a generalized basic entity where the immune status [1] of the patient is altered in such a way that it is more prone for any pathologies involving malignancies, infections, HIV, and fungal infections [2]. With the recent advances in the various imaging modalities where many conditions are being detected in which the immune status of the patent is reduced. Another aspect is the wider use of the medical regimes for various conditions where there is a significant reduction in the immune status. HIV is also an important entity in this lot of conditions, which is caused by the virus [3].

FDG PET is a valuable imaging modality for the diagnosis, staging, detection of metastases, and posttreatment monitoring of several malignancies.

12.1 Introduction

Immunocompromised status is an important pathological entity, which is showing the varied features of loss of immunity. The various causes are of much relevance in this and have important prognostic factors. Since the usefulness of FDG PET is established in various pathologies, immunocompromised status is also an important entity where it is of big help. The commonest causes of immunocompromised status are HIV, metastases, fungal infections, and severe Gram-negative infections. As PET has the ability to differentiate between malignancy and infection in the evaluation of lesions. Immunosuppression predisposes the number of opportunistic infections and therefore special care must be taken while evaluating the PET-CT. Some benign hypermetabolic foci are also giving false-positive results.

© The Author(s), under exclusive license to Springer Nature
Singapore Pte Ltd. 2021
S. Shaikh, *PET-CT in Infection and Inflammation*,
https://doi.org/10.1007/978-981-15-9801-2_12

12.2 HIV

HIV is one of the devastating immunocompromised infections where a significant amount of immunity is lost. The port of entry in HIV is through the mucosal surfaces. Then the virus enters the lymphatic system into the lymph nodes and then into the plasma. The HIV positive effector cells are trapped in the lymph nodes and these lymph nodes are the area for the site of infection [4].

This immunodeficiency is directly proportional to the viral load that is disseminated throughout lymphatic tissues and seen in regional lymph nodes. The pathogenesis is the trapping of HIV positive effector cells in lymphoid tissues, which become reservoirs of viral production [5, 6]. So, lymphocytes activate the glycolysis increasing the glucose uptake in the metabolic areas and the uptake is directly proportional to the amount of activity. HIV patients have varied organ involvement with patterns of lymphoid tissue activation, HIV progression, FDG uptake in head and neck, cervical, axillary and inguinal regions, colon, mesenteric, ileocecal junction, central nervous system, spleen, and various organs [7, 8].

The viremia also plays an important role in the evaluation of immune-compromising infections based on the SUV values. Thus the SUV value is based on the amount of viral load in the body. FDG uptake is directly proportional to the amount of the lymphoid tissue activation and ultimately shows the progression of the disease [9].

12.3 HIV-Related Fungal Infections

Immunocompromised status will lead to many infections, one of the commonest is fungal infections. Fungal infection is also common, especially in the malignant settings of leukemias and especially post-chemotherapy patients. It is associated with impaired cellular immunity in infected patients. HIV-related malignancies are also more commonly seen due to cell-mediated immune deficiency. The commonest entity is Kaposi's sarcoma, lymphoma, epithelial cancer of skin, and various malignancies. In this malignant setting there can be superadded infection due to immunocompromised status involving the T-lymphocytes. Varied presentations of fungal infections in the chest are in the forms of consolidations, cavitation's, fungal ball with or without mediastinal nodes, pleural effusion or pleural thickening, or a combination of these entities. Fungal infections in the neck mostly involving the lymph nodes. CNS's manifestations are seen in various presentations of nodular lesions, ring enhancing lesions, heterogeneously enhancing mass lesions, conglomerate bilobed lesions with significant mass effect, midline shift, perilesional edema, and so many other characteristics findings. These lesions are difficult to distinguish from the primary malignant lesions. However, PET-CT plays an important role only in the form of increased uptake of the lesions. A lot of primary brain tumors have become FDG avid and with new radiotracers like methionine and choline these radiotracers are being used for the primary evaluation, but as far as fungal lesions are concerned FDG PET has a significant role and most of them are sensitive. In the immunocompromised setting, primary lymphoma and variant of Kaposi's sarcoma need to be evaluated. Immunocompromised lesions in the abdomen and pelvis are more prone to infections same as that of other systems. FDG PET has significant role in the evaluation by dual point imaging to differentiate the malignancies and infections as already described. Where it is possible to distinguish between the malignant and infective inflammatory lesions. The neurological manifestations are commonly seen in severely immunocompromised patients with CD4 cell count <200/mm^3. The various opportunistic infections seen are primary CNS lymphoma, toxoplasmosis encephalitis, neurosyphilis, cytomegalovirus encephalitis, tuberculosis, cryptococcosis, progressive multifocal leukoencephalopathy, and CNS lymphoma [10]. Evaluation is based on neurological findings, which is challenging and nonspecific symptoms like fever, headache, altered neurological status, focal or diffuse neurological science, and seizures or it can be a combination of any of these symptoms. Sometimes, FDG uptake is significantly higher than that of nonmalignant lesions. The SUV max values in all these neurological presentations are nonspecific and no significant classical values of a particular pathological entity. However, a definite diagnosis can be made out only by tissue diagnosis (Figs. 12.1 and 12.2).

12.4 HIV and Tuberculosis

The combination of the human immunodeficiency virus and tuberculosis is more severe in the morbidity and mortality. HIV infections usually are more common in the head and neck compared to the chest and abdomen. The FDG uptake is directly proportional to the amount of the viral load and inversely proportional to the CD4 count. FDG PET-CT is not able to clearly distinguish between malignancy and tuberculosis. But another biggest advantage is to evaluate any extrapulmonary infection is there or not. With a single scan of whole-body PET-CT, the concurrent pulmonary and extrapulmonary infections can be identified and thus will help in planning the management.

12.5 HIV-Related Opportunistic Infections

The AIDS-related opportunistic infections are many comprising the bacterial, fungal, viral, and parasitic infections. These infections involve multiple organs and systems.

Pneumocystis carinii pneumonia is one of the most common opportunistic infections in the scenario of AIDS. The hallmark of this infection is CD4 cell count less than 50%. Clinical signs are non-specific, and this PCP organism is not being traced in the culture, so identification is not possible.

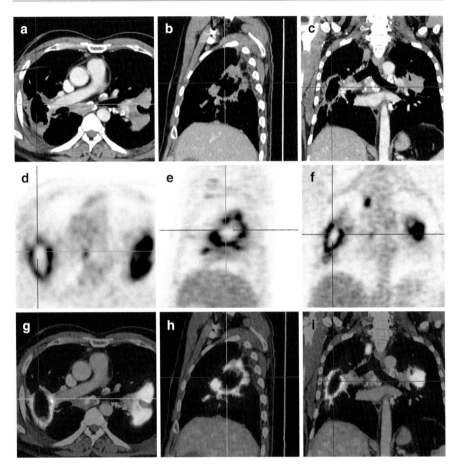

Fig. 12.1 Whole-body PET-CT with CT chest images (**a–c**) showing irregular thick-walled cavity in right lower lobe of lung in CT images with FDG uptake SUV of 4.5 on PET images (**d–f**) and fused images (**g–i**). Another irregular nodular lesion involving left hilar lesion with SUV max of 7.2 consistent with fungal lesions

12.6 Candidiasis

Candidiasis involves mostly the oropharyngeal and esophageal regions. These regions do not show any classical imaging findings. PET-CT though non-specific but plays an important role in this evaluation.

12.7 Immunocompromised Status Human Papilloma Virus Infection

Human papilloma virus-related cancers are more prominently seen in HIV positive patients and associated cervical cancer in women and anal cancers in both male and female. Here FDG PET-CT is increasingly used for staging and evaluation,

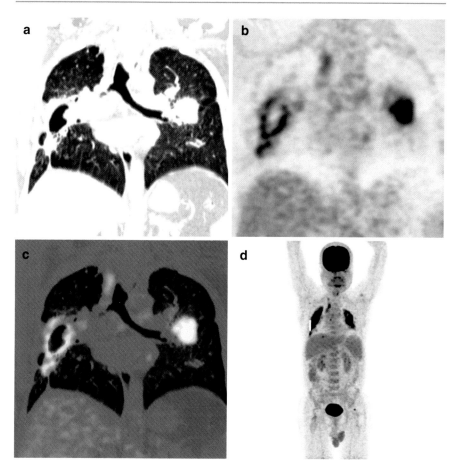

Fig. 12.2 Whole-body PET-CT with CT chest images (**a**) showing irregular thick-walled cavity in right lower lobe of lung in CT images with FDG uptake SUV of 4.5 (**b–d**). Another irregular nodular lesion involving left hilar lesion with SUV max of 7.2 consistent with fungal lesions

recurrence, predicting outcome, and post-therapy evaluation. Here the basis is immunocompromised status.

Human papilloma-related cancers are frequently seen in HIV positive patients. In this, there is an increased risk of cervical cancer in females and anal carcinomas in males and females. Here the role of the evaluation is based on the various factors like staging, restaging, and monitoring response to the treatment.

12.8   HIV-Related Malignancies

HIV infection as known has impaired cellular immunity leading to the development of the neoplasms. This also has some relevance in relation to the organ transplant recipients, immunosuppressive therapy, and cell-mediated immune deficiencies. The tumors associated with the HICV are Kaposi's sarcoma, lymphomas, skin cancers, and anogenital malignancies [11–14]. The viruses associated with HIV are Epstein-Barr virus and Herpes simplex virus.

12.9 Lymphoma

Lymphoma is one of the commonest pathologies in immunosuppressive disorders, which are Non-Hodgkin's Lymphoma [15]. The different features involved in all this are Burkitt's lymphoma, diffuse large B cell lymphoma with centroblastic features. Burkitt's lymphoma is the commonest lymphoma in HIV FDG PET-CT is the important modality for imaging [16] (Figs. 12.3, 12.4, 12.5, and 12.6).

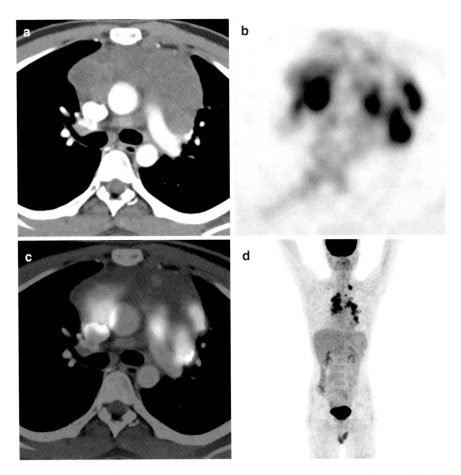

Fig. 12.3 Whole-body PET-CT CT image (**a**) showing patchily enhancing anterior mediastinal mass showing inhomogeneous enhancement and significant metabolic activity in PET images (**b**, **d**) and fused image (**c**) with SUV max of 7.9 suggestive of mediastinal lymphoma

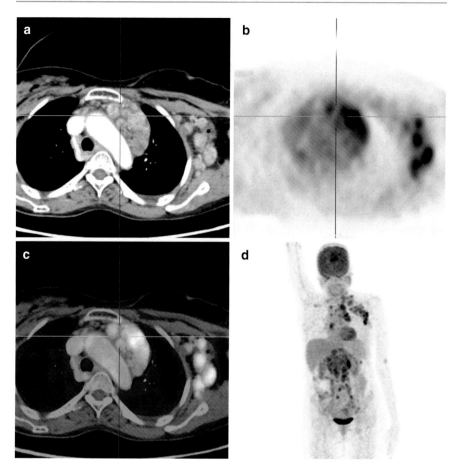

Fig. 12.4 Whole-body PET-CT CT, CT images showing multiple conglomerates in homoge-nously enhancing metabolically active lymph nodes in fused and PET images in anterior medias-tinum, left axilla, abdomen, and pelvis with significant metabolic activity with SUV max of 7.7. Findings suggestive of tuberculosis

12.10   CNS Infections in HIV

Neurological complications are seen more commonly in HIV positive patients due to many opportunistic infections, associated malignancies, and HIV infections itself. The amount of immune suppression is the important factor in this evaluation. The various infections involving the s are Toxoplasmosis, Neurosyphilis, Cytomegalovirus encephalitis, Tuberculosis, Cryptococcosis, Progressive multifo-cal leukoencephalopathy and primary CNS Lymphomas. PET-CT plays an impor-tant role in the evaluation but not able to differentiate between the two different pathological entities [10, 17–19].

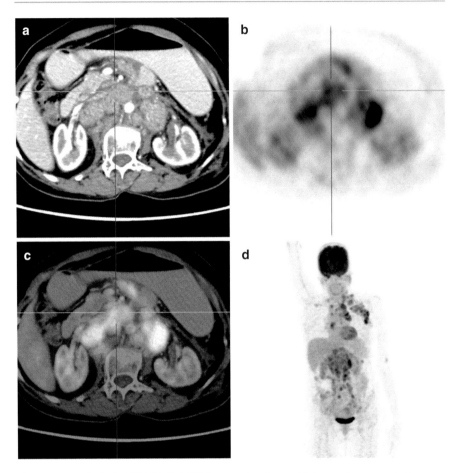

Fig. 12.5 Whole-body PET-CT CT, CT images showing multiple conglomerates in homoge-nously enhancing metabolically active lymph nodes in fused and PET images in anterior medias-tinum, left axilla, abdomen, and pelvis with significant metabolic activity with SUV max of 7.7. Findings suggestive of tuberculosis

12.11 Fever of Unknown Origin

Immunosuppression due to HIV infections is the predisposing factor for various opportunistic infections. Here the role of FDG PET-CT is to locate the site of infection and the extent of the infection. Thus, FDG PET-CT plays an important role in the evaluation of the HIV-related various causes of fever of unknown origin [20].

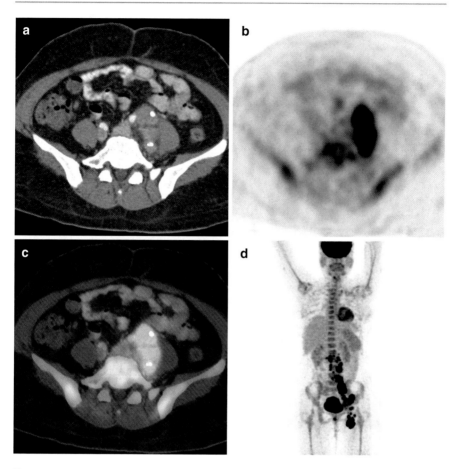

Fig. 12.6 Whole-body PET-CT CT, CT images showing multiple conglomerates in homogenously enhancing metabolically active lymph nodes in fused and PET images in anterior mediastinum, left axilla, abdomen, and pelvis with significant metabolic activity with SUV max of 7.7. Findings suggestive of tuberculosis

12.12 Post-immunotherapy Evaluation

The mainline treatment of autoimmune diseases is highly active antiretroviral therapy (HAART). FDG PET is useful in evaluating the response to therapy in the settings of HAART therapy. It also helps in signifying the associated morbidity and mortality in this therapy. Few of the patients who do not respond to this HAART therapy arc known as immune reconstitution inflammatory syndrome [21, 22]. Patients with this syndrome show clinical deterioration due to the development of opportunistic infection symptoms like tuberculosis, herpes simplex virus, toxoplasmosis, and bacterial pneumonia. One of the diagnostic features of this immune reconstitution inflammatory syndrome is new lymph nodes or enlargement of the nodes in the existing conditions. One of the important side effects of HAART is lipodystrophy where there is peripheral wasting of fat central adiposity and metabolic changes such as hyperlipidemia, hyperglycemia, and insulin resistance.

Evaluation of PET for other associated infections and inflammations in relation to esophagus and oropharynx. It also helps in the evaluation of generalized lymphadenopathy and distinct forms of lymphoid tissue activation. The basis of this is the viral load and low CD4 T-cell counts. With the excellent biodistribution of FDG uptake is seen as lymphoid tissue activation and provides valuable information about the status of the disease. FDG PET has proven useful in the diagnosis staging, monitoring response to therapy, and any association with metastases. The era of HAART has brought significant changes in the management of HIV positive patients and PET plays an important role not only in the criteria mentioned above but also in evaluation of various side effects as lipodystrophy. With these, new antiretroviral regimes can be developed in the future.

12.13 Immunosuppressive Drugs and Antiretroviral Therapy

Immunosuppressive drugs and antiretroviral therapy are the mainstay treatment for HIV patients. Significant impact is noted on the lesions involved by HIV and also on the other systems of the body. This antiretroviral therapy has blend of effects and FDG PET-CT is helpful in the evaluation of monitoring response to therapy [23–25].

Immunosuppressive drugs affect the metabolism of leukocytes and also FDG uptake in inflamed tissue. This only anticipated and desired effect having an impact on the diagnosis of various diseases where corticosteroid is used for treatment. FDG PET is altered by the sensitivity and not the specificity of corticosteroid therapy. One of the important criteria for accurate diagnosis of inflammatory diseases by FDG PET is to temporarily withhold the immunosuppressive therapy by 2 weeks as per the guidelines recommended by the European Association of Nuclear Medicine (EANM).

12.14 Conclusion

FDG PET-CT plays an important role in the evaluation of blend of pathologies in HIV patients. Dual time point imaging is helpful to differentiate between malignant and various infective and inflammatory pathologies.

References

1. Niu MT, Jermano JA, Reichelderfer P, Schnittman SM. Summary of the National Institutes of Health workshop on primary human immunodeficiency virus type 1 infection. AIDS Res Hum Retroviruses. 1993;9:913–24.

2. [No authors listed]. UNAIDS 2008 report on the global AIDS epidemic. Joint United Nations Programme on HIV/AIDS. www.unaids.org/en/dataanalysis/epidemiology/2008reportonthegl obalaidsepidemic. Published July 29, 2008. Accessed 7 April 2011.

3. Fox CH, Tenner-Racz K, Racz P, Firpo A, Pizzo PA, Fauci AS. Lymphoid germinal centers are reservoirs of human immunodeficiency virus type 1 RNA. J Infect Dis. 1991;164:1051–7.

4. Pantaleo G, Graziosi C, Demarest JF, et al. Role of lymphoid organs in the pathogenesis of human immunodeficiency virus (HIV) infection. Immunol Rev. 1994;140:105–30.

5. Tenner-Racz K, Racz P, Gluckman JC, Popovic M. Cell-free HIV in lymph nodes of patients with AIDS and generalized lymphadenopathy. N Engl J Med. 1988;318:49–50.

6. Pantaleo G, Graziosi C, Butini L, et al. Lymphoid organs function as major reservoirs for human immunodeficiency virus. Proc Natl Acad Sci USA. 1991;88:9838–42.

7. Bakheet SM, Powe J. Benign causes of 18-FDG uptake on whole body imaging. Semin Nucl Med. 1998;28:352–8.

8. Sugawara Y, Braun DK, Kison PV, Russo JE, Zasadny KR, Wahl RL. Rapid detection of human infections with fluorine-18 fluorodeoxyglucose and positron emission tomography: preliminary results. Eur J Nucl Med. 1998;25:1238–43.

9. Brust D, Polis M, Davey R, et al. Fluorodeoxyglucose imaging in healthy subjects with HIV infection: impact of disease stage and therapy on pattern of nodal activation. AIDS. 2006;20:985–93.

10. Manzardo C, Del Mar OM, Sued O, Garcia F, Moreno A, Miro JM. Central nervous system opportunistic infections in developed countries in the highly active antiretroviral therapy era. J Neurovirol. 2005;11(Suppl 3):72–82.

11. Smith EM, Ritchie JM, Summersgill KF, et al. Human papilloma virus in oral exfoliated cells and risk of head and neck cancer. J Natl Cancer Inst. 2004;96:449–55.

12. Sathekge M, Maes A, Al-Nahhas A, Rubello D, Chiti A. What impact can fluorine-18 fluorode-oxyglucose PET/computed tomography have on HIV/AIDS and tuberculosis pandemic? Nucl Med Commun. 2009;30:255–7.

13. Cotter SE, Grigsby PW, Siegel BA, et al. FDG-PET/CT in the evaluation of anal carcinoma. Int J Radiat Oncol Biol Phys. 2006;65:720–5.

14. DeMario MD, Liebowitz DN. Lymphomas in the immune-compromised patient. Semin Oncol. 1998;25:492–502.

15. Goshen E, Davidson T, Avigdor A, Zwas TS, Levy I. PET/CT in the evaluation of lymphoma in patients with HIV-1 with suppressed viral loads. Clin Nucl Med. 2008;33:610–4.

16. Hoffman JM, Waskin HA, Schifter T, et al. FDG-PET in differentiating lymphoma from non-malignant central nervous system lesions in patients with AIDS. J Nucl Med. 1993;34:567–75.

17. Carbone A, Gloghini A. AIDS-related lymphomas: from pathogenesis to pathology. Br J Haematol. 2005;130:662–70.

18. Just PA, Fieschi C, Baillet G, Galicier L, Oksenhendler E, Moretti JL. 18F-fluorodeoxyglucose positron emission tomography/computed tomography in AIDS-related Burkitt lymphoma. AIDS Patient Care STDs. 2008;22:695–700.

19. Villringer K, Jager H, Dichgans M, et al. Differential diagnosis of CNS lesions in AIDS patients by FDG-PET. J Comput Assist Tomogr. 1995;19:532–6.

20. Heald AE, Hoffman JM, Bartlett JA, Waskin HA. Differentiation of central nervous system lesions in AIDS patients using positron emission tomography (PET). Int J STD AIDS. 1996;7:337–46.

21. Kwan A, Seltzer M, Czernin J, Chou MJ, Kao CH. Characterization of hilar lymphnode by 18F-fluoro-2-deoxyglucose positron emission tomography in healthy subjects. Anticancer Res. 2001;21:701–6.

22. Castaigne C, Tondeur M, de Wit S, Hildebrand M, Clumeck N, Dusart M. Clinical value of FDG-PET/CT for the diagnosis of human immunodeficiency virus-associated fever of unknown origin: a retrospective study. Nucl Med Commun. 2009;30:41–7.

23. Nasti G, Talamini R, Antinori A, et al. AIDS-related Kaposi's sarcoma: evaluation of potential new prognostic factors and assessment of the AIDS clinical trial group staging system in the HAART era—the Italian Cooperative Group on AIDS and tumors and the Italian cohort of patients naive from antiretrovirals. J Clin Oncol. 2003;21:2876–82.

24. Rubio A, Martinez-Moya M, Leal M, et al. Changes in thymus volume in adult HIV-infected patients under HAART: correlation with the T-cell repopulation. Clin Exp Immunol. 2002;130:121–6.
25. Bower M, Palmieri C, Dhillon T. AIDS-related malignancies: changing epidemiology and the impact of highly active antiretroviral therapy. Curr Opin Infect Dis. 2006;19:14–9.

PET-CT in Polymyalgia Rheumatica

13

Key Points

Polymyalgia Rheumatica is an important inflammatory disorder, which is common in the elderly with inflammatory changes. This is associated with vasculitis like giant cell arteritis and rheumatoid arthritis. Polymyalgia Rheumatica is diagnosed based on clinical and inflammatory findings.

FDG PET is an important modality for the diagnosis of polymyalgia. There can be various other associated features.

13.1 Introduction

Polymyalgia Rheumatica is an inflammatory disorder common in over 50 years of age and with common symptoms like neck pain, shoulder pain, hip pain, morning stiffness, and associated with increased inflammatory parameters [1, 2]. Polymyalgia Rheumatica can coexist with giant cell arteritis or rheumatoid arthritis or isolated phenomenon [3]. Glucocorticoids are the drug of choice and show a good response. However, this response to glucocorticoids is non-specific. The clinical diagnosis can be made by the pain and stiffness involving the joint more than the 30 min and aggravating after the rest. Absence of Rheumatoid factor or any other joint involvement is also another criterion. This is seen more commonly in the shoulder, neck, and hip joints. Pain is usually sudden starting unilaterally initially but later on, it becomes bilateral. The constitutional symptoms are fatigue, malaise, anorexia, depression, weight loss, and more commonly low-grade fever. The peripheral joints are less commonly involved, and the involvement is in the form of symmetrical arthritis commonly involving the knee, wrists, and small joints of the hand. Common differential diagnosis is nonerosive metacarpophalangeal and proximal interphalangeal arthritis, which needs further early evaluation. Swelling and edema of the hands and feet due to tenosynovitis is the first presenting symptom. Examinations should also include evaluation of the temporal arteries, peripheral pulses, and

S. Shaikh, *PET-CT in Infection and Inflammation*,
https://doi.org/10.1007/978-981-15-9801-2_13

auscultation for bruits. If vascular abnormalities are present then further evaluation of the GCA should be undertaken. Imaging of blood vessels in patients with PMR shows findings of vasculitis even in patients without signs and symptoms.

13.2   Criteria for Evaluation of Polymyalgia Rheumatica

Polymyalgia Rheumatica can be assessed by increased C-reactive protein (CRP) level or Erythrocyte Sedimentation Rate (ESR), and onset of hip pain. The sensitivity and specificity of these criterias were 68% and 78%, respectively. FDG PET scan diagnosed precisely. FDG avidity is focused more common around the shoulders, hips, and spinous process of lumbar or cervical vertebrae. Yamashita and colleagues [4] performed FDG PET-CT in 14 patients with untreated active PMR and 17 control patients with rheumatoid arthritis and other rheumatic diseases. They demonstrated a similar involvement in the sternoclavicular joints, ischial tuberosities, greater trochanters, and spinous processes. As glucocorticoid is an important line of management, FDG PET plays important role in the pre- and post-therapy evaluations.

One of the criteria is the total skeletal score which can be calculated with the clinical suspicion of PMR and visualized score in 12 different articular regions, shoulders, hips, sternoclavicular joints, ischial tuberosities, greater trochanters, cervical spinous process, and lumbar processes. With this criterion, the diagnosis of PMR is done taking into consideration all the aspects of clinical data, biochemical data, sensitivity, specificity, positive predictive value, negative predictive value, and total skeletal score.

13.3   Role of FDG PET-CT in the Polymyalgia Rheumatica

Positron emission tomography (PET) is an important imaging modality for the evaluation of Polymyalgia Rheumatica. Fluorodeoxyglucose (FDG) uptake is commonly seen in the shoulders, hips, and the cervical and lumbar interspinous processes of patients with PMR. The vascular inflammation is also seen commonly in this condition and helps in the evaluation of PMR.

FDG PET plays an important role in the pre- and post-therapy evaluations of glucocorticoid therapy. This is usually done at 3 and 6 months after the therapy to evaluate the response to treatment. At this time, the disease can be asymptomatic and laboratory findings may be normal in most of the cases [5, 6] (Fig. 13.1).

13.4   Role of FDG PET-CT in Assessing Large Cell Vasculitis
         in Polymyalgia Rheumatica

Polymyalgia Rheumatica is commonly associated with large cell vasculitis in 21% of patients [7–9]. The relapse of Polymyalgia Rheumatica is also there and common. FDG PET usually having a correlation with the symptoms or elevated levels

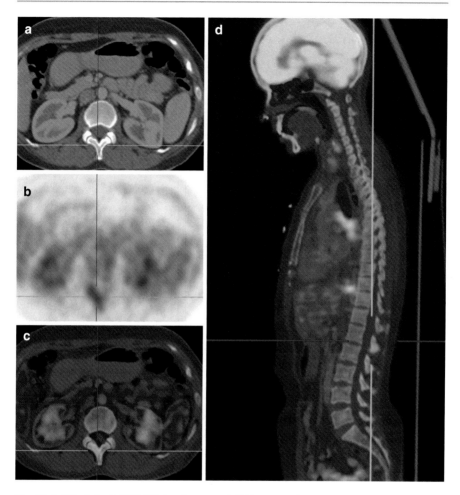

Fig. 13.1 Whole-body PET-CT showing normal CT image (**a**) fused image (**c, d**) and PET image (**b**) showing mild uptake along the spinous process of L1 vertebral body features consistent with polymyalgia

of acute-phase proteins and other symptomatic clinical findings. The large- and medium-sized vessel vasculitis are also common and shows the inflammatory changes of the external carotid branches, including temporal and occipital arteries, the ophthalmic, vertebral, distal subclavian, and axillary arteries. The symptoms suggestive of vasculitis are new-onset headache, jaw claudication, scalp tenderness, visual disorders, carotidynia, and limb claudication are common in the PMR and need to undergo confirmation testing the diagnostic testing to evaluate associated GCA.

13.5   Role of FDG PET-CT in Differential Diagnosis of Polymyalgia Rheumatica and Rheumatoid Arthritis

FDG PET plays an important role in distinguishing Polymyalgia Rheumatica and rheumatoid arthritis. Basis of evaluation is the higher metabolic activity in PMR sites compared with rheumatoid arthritis [10–18]. Other points of differentiation with rheumatoid arthritis which shows increased uptake at the enthesis of muscles and other locations like cervical and lumbar vertebrae, ischial tuberosity, greater trochanter, and shoulder joints. Wakura and colleagues [19] compared abnormal FDG uptake and by the above evaluation criteria, FDG PET-CT is useful in differentiating PMR from early RA.

Many conditions mimic PMR and should be evaluated and differentiated in the diagnostic approach of the patients with proximal inflammatory muscular pain and stiffness. Clinical history and physical examination are important in distinguishing PMR from other conditions. These conditions which can be differentiated are inflammatory and noninflammatory musculoskeletal disorders, infectious diseases, endocrinopathies, malignancies, and other disorders like hypovitaminosis D, depression, and drug-induced myopathy. The other differential diagnoses are spondyloarthritis, vasculitis, connective tissue disorders, inflammatory arthritis, crystalline myositis, degenerative joint disease, fibromyalgia, thyroid disorders, infections, and many more conditions (Figs. 13.2, 13.3, and 13.4).

13.6   Polymyalgia Rheumatica and Associated Cardiovascular Involvement

Inflammatory and autoimmune pathologies show more chances of cardiovascular risks. Various factors can be used to evaluate these risk factors. The various CV risk factors, chronic inflammation, and autoimmune system dysregulation are important in the induction and progression of atherosclerotic vascular damage. The imbalance between endothelial micro-particle (EMP) release and endothelial progenitor cell (EPC) generation is demonstrated. Various markers of endothelial injury, CV risk, and metabolic risk factors in the general population plays an important role. The basic and main mechanism is the underlying vascular damage in PMR, which can cause endothelial dysfunction, damage due to the systemic inflammatory burden of the disease, and the association of PMR with inflammatory arteritis (GCA). Long-term glucocorticoid treatment should also be considered an important factor for CV damage in patients with PMR. GC therapy with high doses may cause harmful CV effects by increasing the risk due to effects on lipids, glucose tolerance, weight gain, and hypertension [20–23].

The important regulatory factor of inflammatory cell infiltration in the vessel wall, thrombus formation, and smooth muscle cell proliferation is important.

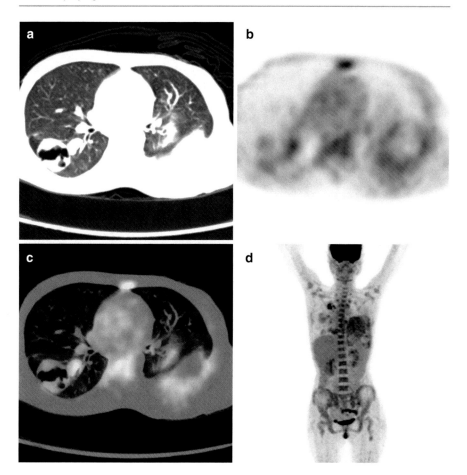

Fig. 13.2 Whole-body PET-CT with chest sections CT image (**a**) showing nodular lesion with cavitation in right lower lobe and PET images (**b, d**) and fused image (**c**) showing significant metabolic activity with SUV max of 6.5. Findings suggestive of connective tissue lesions

Endothelial layer reparative ability is maintained by EPC's ability to form new blood vessels through a process of vasculogenesis by homing on sites of vascular injury.

There is an increased systemic risk of atherosclerosis that can be seen associated with systemic inflammations, autoimmune inflammation, and chronic inflammations which can be seen as the elevated inflammatory biomarkers. Inflammatory arteritis is also seen in association with cardiac involvement. The various predisposing cardiac factors are also seen in this association. PET-CT is important modality for the evaluation of the various cardiac and vascular pathologies (Fig. 13.5).

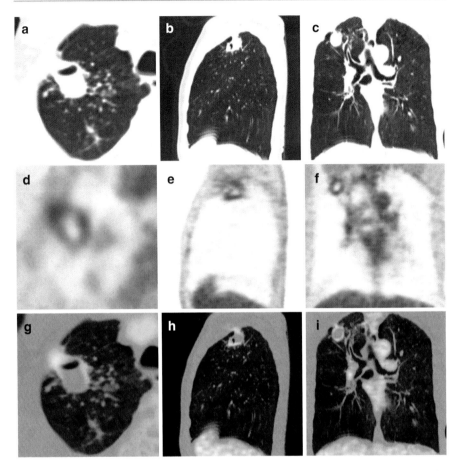

Fig. 13.3 Whole-body PET-CT with chest sections CT image (**a**) showing nodular lesion with cavitation in right lower lobe and PET images (**b, d**) and fused image (**c**) showing significant metabolic activity with SUV max of 6.5. Findings suggestive of connective tissue lesions

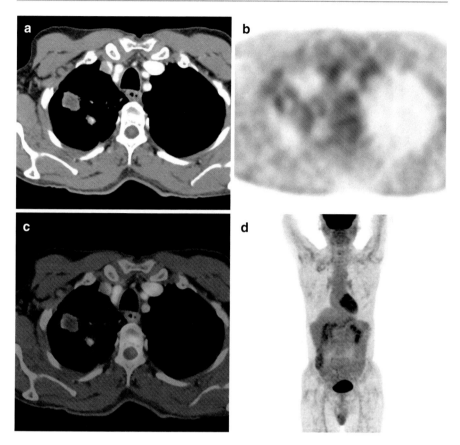

Fig. 13.4 Whole-body PET-CT at the level of chest, CT image (**a**) showing nodule in right upper lobe with minimal uptake in fused image (**c**) and PET images (**b**, **d**) suggestive of collage disease

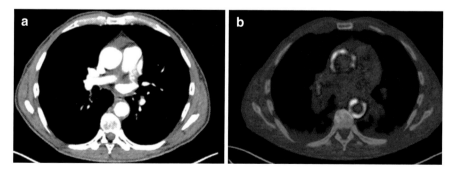

Fig. 13.5 Diffuse circumferential wall thickening seen in ascending and descending thoracic aorta in CT image (**a**) with diffuse circumferential uptake in PET image (**b**) with SUV max of 4.0 suggestive of vasculitis associated with Polymyalgia Rheumatica

13.7   Conclusion

Thus, FDG PET-CT plays a significant role in the evaluation of Polymyalgia
Rheumatica to differentiate between different conditions and also to monitor the
response to therapy.

References

1. Calabrese C, Cappelli LC, Kostine M, et al. Polymyalgia rheumatica-like syndrome from checkpoint inhibitor therapy: case series and systematic review of the literature. RMD Open. 2019;5:e000906.
2. Kostine M, Rouxel L, Barnetche T, et al. Rheumatic disorders associated with immune checkpoint inhibitors in patients with cancer-clinical aspects and relationship with tumour response: a single-centre prospective cohort study. Ann Rheum Dis. 2018;77:393–8.
3. Kermani T, Warrington K. Polymyalgia rheumatica. Lancet. 2013;381:63–72.
4. Yamashita H, Kubota K, Takahashi Y, Minamimoto R, Morooka M, Kaneko H, Kano T, Mimori A. Similarities and differences in fluorodeoxyglucose positron emission tomography/computed tomography findings in spondyloarthropathy, polymyalgia rheumatica and rheumatoid arthritis. Joint Bone Spine. 2013;80:171–7. https://doi.org/10.1016/j.jbspin.2012.04.006.
5. Jaruskova M, Belohlavek O. Role of FDG-PET and PET/CT in the diagnosis of prolonged febrile states. Eur J Nucl Med Mol Imaging. 2006;33:913–8. https://doi.org/10.1007/s00259-006-0064-z.
6. Kubota K, Nakamoto Y, Tamaki N, Kanegae K, Fukuda H, Kaneda T, et al. FDGPET for the diagnosis of fever of unknown origin: a Japanese multi-center study. Ann Nucl Med. 2011;25:355–64. https://doi.org/10.1007/s12149-011-0470-6.
7. Lensen KDF, Comans EFI, Voskuyl AE, Van der Laken CJ, Brouwer E, Zwijnenburg AT, et al. Large-vessel vasculitis: interobserver agreement and diagnostic accuracy of 18 F-FDG-PET/CT. Biomed Res Int. 2015; https://doi.org/10.1155/2015/914692.
8. Fuchs M, Briel M, Daikeler T, Walker UA, Rasch H, Berg S, et al. The impact of 18F-FDG PET on the management of patients with suspected large vessel vasculitis. Eur J Nucl Med Mol Imaging. 2012;39:344–53. https://doi.org/10.1007/s00259-011-1967-x.
9. Taniguchi Y, Nakayama S, Terada Y. Clinical implication of FDG-PET/CT in monitoring disease activity in large-vessel giant cell arteritis linked with secondary polymyalgia rheumatica. Case Rep Internal Med. 2014;1:6–9. https://doi.org/10.5430/crim.v1n1p6.
10. Ruta S, Rosa J, Navarta DA, Saucedo C, Catoggio LJ, Monaco RG, et al. Ultrasound assessment of new onset bilateral painful shoulder in patients with polymyalgia rheumatica and rheumatoid arthritis. Clin Rheumatol. 2012;31:1383–7. https://doi.org/10.1007/s10067-012-2016-2.
11. Henckaerts L, Gheysens O, Blockmans D. Use of 18F-fluorodeoxyglucose positron emission tomography in the diagnosis of polymyalgia rheumatic – a prospective study of 99 patients. Rheumatology. 2017;57(11):1908–16.
12. Clifford A, Cimmino M. In search of a diagnostic test for polymyalgia rheumatica: is positron emission tomography the answer? Rheumatology. 2018;57:1881–2.
13. Jones JG, Hazleman BL. Prognosis and management of polymyalgia rheumatica. Ann Rheum Dis. 1981;40:1–5. https://doi.org/10.1136/ard.40.1.1.
14. Blockmans D, De Ceuninck L, Vanderschueren S, Knockaert D, Mortelmans L, Bobbaers H. Repetitive 18-fluorodeoxyglucose positron emission tomography in isolated polymyalgia rheumatica: a prospective study in 35 patients. Rheumatology. 2007;46:672–7. https://doi.org/10.1093/rheumatology/kel376.
15. Rehak Z, Vasina J, Nemec P, Fojtik Z, Koukalova R, Bortlicek Z, et al. Various forms of 18F-FDG PET and PET/CT findings in patients with polymyalgia rheumatica. Biomed Pap

Med Fac Univ Palacky Olomouc Czech Repub. 2015;159:629–36. https://doi.org/10.5507/bp.2015.026.

16. Toriihara A, Seto Y, Yoshida K, Umehara I, Nakagawa T, Tassei MD, et al. F-18 FDG PET/CT of polymyalgia rheumatica. Clin Nucl Med. 2009;34:305–6. https://doi.org/10.1097/RLU.0b013e31819e51fd.

17. Kotani T, Komori T, Kanzaki Y, Takeuchi T, Wakura D, Iimori A, et al. FDGPET/CT of polymyalgia rheumatica. Mod Rheumatol. 2011;21:334–6. https://doi.org/10.1007/s10165-010-0382-7.

18. Park JS, Pyo JY, Park HJ, Lee HS, Kang Y, Kang MI, et al. Typical 18-FDG-PET/CT findings of polymyalgia rheumatica: a case report. J Rheumatic Dis. 2013;20:113–7. https://doi.org/10.4078/jrd.2013.20.2.113.

19. Wakura D, Kotani T, Takeuchi T, Komori T, Yoshida S, Makino S, et al. Differentiation between polymyalgia Rheumatica (PMR) and elderly-onset rheumatoid arthritis using 18F-fluorodeoxyglucose positron emission tomography/computed tomography: is enthesitis a new pathological lesion in PMR? PLoS One. 2016;11:e0158509. https://doi.org/10.1371/journal.pone.0158509.

20. Bartoloni E, et al. Inflammatory and autoimmune mechanisms in the induction of atherosclerotic damage in systemic rheumatic diseases: two faces of the same coin. Arthritis Care Res. 2011;63:178–83.

21. Olsson A, Elling H, Elling P. Frequency of a normal erythrocyte sedimentation rate in patients with active, untreated arteritis temporalis and polymyalgia rheumatica: comment on the article by Helfgott and Kieval. Arthritis Rheum. 1997;40:191–3.

22. Burger D, et al. Cellular biomarkers of endothelial health: micro-particles, endothelial progenitor cells, and circulating endothelial cells. J Am Soc Hypertens. 2012;6:85–99.

23. Amabile N, et al. Association of circulating endothelial micro-particles with cardiometabolic risk factors in the Framingham Heart Study. Eur Heart J. 2014;35:2972–9.

PET-CT in Pediatric Infection and Inflammation

14

Key Points

Fever of unknown origin and associated signs of inflammation are one of the most challenging medical conditions in pediatric age group. The associated laboratory findings, demographic parameters, and clinical findings do not have any relevance in pediatric age group. This diagnostic approach is mostly non-specific comprising clinical examination, laboratory tests, radiological procedures, and other invasive tests like biopsy, bone marrow examination, and others. Many routine modalities like conventional radiography, Ultrasound, Doppler, CT, MRI, and Nuclear studies are being done for various indications related to the fever of unknown origin. FDG PET-CT is the newer imaging modality for the evaluation of various pathologies related to the infective and inflammatory diseases PET-CT in pediatrics has to be followed under the principle of ALARA.

14.1 Introduction

Fever of unknown origin is one of the most important clinical entities, which is challenging and has various causes ranging from malignancies, infections, autoimmune diseases, and other noninfectious inflammatory pathologies. As already mentioned, the definition of FUO is temperature higher than 38.3^0 on various occasions, which lasts more than 3 weeks and where the diagnosis is not certain after admission to the hospital at least for a week [1]. The diagnosis of FUO is extensive and cumbersome which includes physical examination, laboratory tests, radiological imaging, and invasive procedures like biopsy and bone marrow. This is important because as per the literature the causes of FUO are more than 200. Tuberculosis is the most common cause of FUO in developing countries. In pediatric age group, FUO etiology rate is more than 56.7% and it mostly represents as localized infections. Rheumatoid arthritis is one of the important causes. This evaluation of FUO is sometimes

© The Author(s), under exclusive license to Springer Nature
Singapore Pte Ltd. 2021
S. Shaikh, *PET-CT in Infection and Inflammation*,
https://doi.org/10.1007/978-981-15-9801-2_14

traumatic to the child and may prolong the diagnosis resulting in various changes in the growth and development of a child. With this background, the early diagnosis of FUO in the children is important with a single modality, which can define this. Thus, FDG PET-CT has become the gold standard for diagnostic workup of FUO [2–6].

FDG PET-CT has been established and plays important role in nonmalignant and benign pediatric pathologies [7, 8]. Infection inflammation the most common cause of nonmalignant conditions and needs to be used cautiously due to the amount of the radiation involved in this whole-body scan.

With the advent of FDG PET-CT in oncologic practice, a lot of coexisting nonmalignant pathologies are also detected incidentally. Few of these pathologies are concurrent and few of them are the result of post-therapy complications. F-FDG is the most commonly used radiotracer for PET and demonstrates the metabolic activity proportionate to the amount of the disease activity. FDG accumulates in tumor cells as well as proliferating inflammatory cells granulocytes, monocytes, and lymphocytes. Thus, with this imaging of acute as well chronic inflammatory pathology evaluation is easier. FDG PET functional activity of inflammation directly proportional to the amount of inflammatory activity [3, 9]. The basic principle is same in FDG PET-CT for the evaluation of the disease activity.

14.2 Pathophysiology of Infection and Inflammation

The important indication for FDG PET in pediatric age group is oncological indications. However, it is being widely used for the infective and inflammatory conditions. The stimulus of septic focus is the mechanism initiated by the release of local chemokines, interleukins (ILs), and prostaglandins that are well known proinflammatory mediators [10, 11].

Abudised et al. [12] demonstrated a high accumulation of macrophages and granulation tissues in animal models in the access. Thus, increased uptake is seen in the inflammatory cells like granulocytes, leukocytes, and macrophages at the entry. In this scenario, FDG PET is active throughout the lungs including the interstitium. FDG PET-CT, The normal sites of physiological uptakes needs to be kept in mind like spleen, bone marrow and bowel activity [13].

14.3 Detection of FUO

Many imaging methods are used for the diagnosis of FUO. The commonly used are Ga-68 citrate scan [14], labeled leukocyte scan (Tc-99m, In-111), labeled immunoglobulin scan (Tc-99m or In-111) FDG PET-CT, and WBC PET-CT scans [15, 16]. Labeled immunoglobulin scan is used for the diagnosis of infection and inflammation. The advantage of radiolabeled monoclonal antibodies against surface antigens or granulocytes is easier.

14.4   Neurological Infections

Neurological infections are the important clinical conditions that can be diagnosed by PET-CT depending on the amount of FDG uptake and SUV values. The amount of uptake is directly proportional to the amount of glycolysis in the particular tissue. Meningitis and encephalitis are the important causes of neurological involvement by infections. The causes are varied from infection caused by bacteria, viral, fungal, parasitic, and various nonmalignant causes. This has to be differentiated from the malignant FDG uptake [17] (Fig. 14.1).

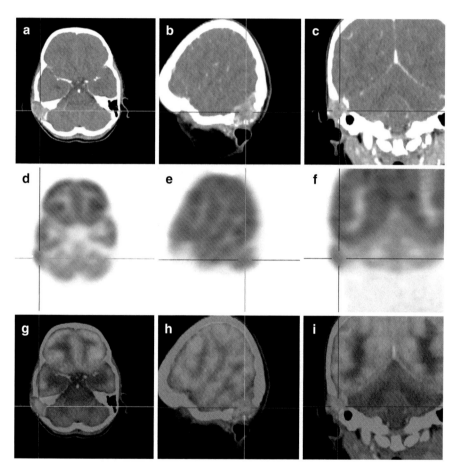

Fig. 14.1   PET-CT brain CT images (**a–c**) showing patchily enhancing soft tissue with erosion of the right mastoid with minimal FDG uptake seen in PET images (**d–f**) and fused images (**g–i**) with SUV max of 1.5 suggestive of right mastoiditis

14.5   FDG Uptake in Head and Neck

The common cause of pediatric infections in head and neck are infective inflammatory pathologies involving the Waldeyers ring comprising of tonsils and the lymphoid tissue. Nasopharynx is also the important cause which needs to be evaluated. The other clinical entities are parotitis, sialadenitis, sinusitis, and thyroiditis. Here the role of FDG PET-CT is to evaluate the tentative cause based on the amount of FDG uptake in various tissues [18, 19] (Figs. 14.2 and 14.3).

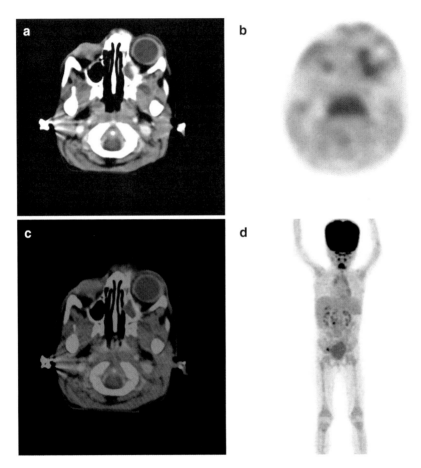

Fig. 14.2 Whole-body PET-CT CT image showing focal soft tissue prominence in nasopharynx with mild FDG uptake of 2.8 in PET and fused images in the nasopharynx suggestive of infective inflammatory pathology

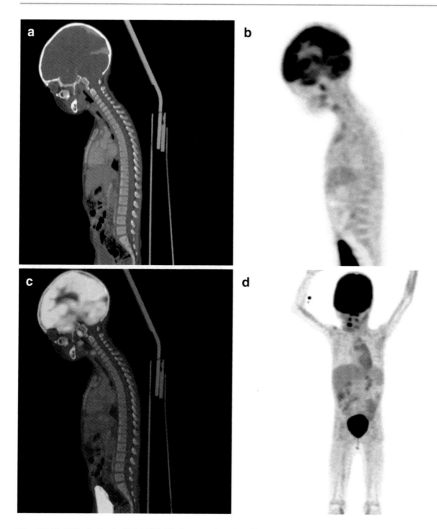

Fig. 14.3 Whole-body PET-CT CT image showing focal soft tissue prominence in nasopharynx with mild FDG uptake of 2.8 in PET and fused images in the nasopharynx suggestive of infective inflammatory pathology

14.6   Chest

Chest infections are an important cause now of FUO. Various chest infections like tuberculosis, bacterial, and viral causes are important ones. Differentiation with the malignant pathologies needs to be differentiated. Mediastinal causes like mediastinitis, pleura, and chest wall are also important for the differentiation. The amount of FDG uptake is directly proportional to the amount of disease involvement [20]. SUV max plays an important role in the evaluation and to distinguish

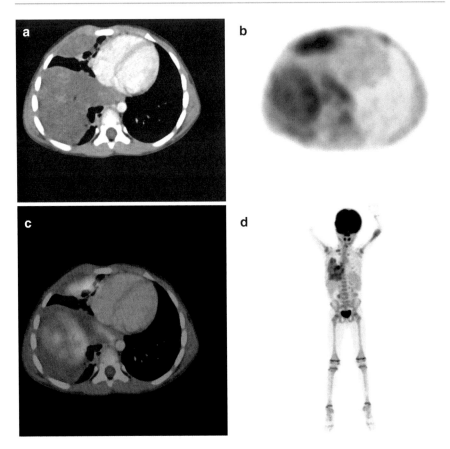

Fig. 14.4 Whole-body PET-CT CT image showing moderate right pleural effusion with collapse of the lung and nodular pleural thickening showing diffuse increased uptake with SUV max of 4.2. Bilateral uptake noted in epiphysis of shoulder, elbow, hip, knee, and ankle

between malignant and infective inflammatory pathologies by dual point time delayed imaging [21]. The more the active lesion more the SUV max value (Fig. 14.4 and 14.5).

14.6.1 Cystic Fibrosis

The basic pathophysiology is predominantly inflammatory cells that secrets pro-inflammatory mediators, releasing patent proteases. The FDG uptake in cystic fibrosis based on the associated inflammation which is more prominent in apical portions of the lung. PET also helps in monitoring airway inflammation, diagnosing anti-inflammatory effects, and response to therapy evaluation. Ideally, PET is not the first line of diagnosis for cystic fibrosis. But with recent advancements, PET is playing an important role in the evaluation of these lesions [22].

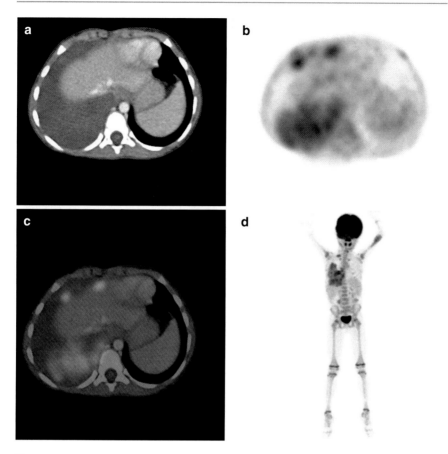

Fig. 14.5 Whole-body PET-CT CT image showing moderate right pleural effusion with collapse of the lung and nodular pleural thickening showing diffuse increased uptake with SUV max of 4.2. Bilateral uptake noted in epiphysis of shoulder, elbow, hip, knee, and ankle

14.6.2 Acute Respiratory Distress Syndrome

Acute Respiratory Distress Syndrome (ARDS) is an important clinical entity that is associated with acute lung injury and a lot of inflammatory processes and mechanisms. There are significant morbidity and mortality in critically ill patients. The basis of FDG PET imaging is to potentially give quantitative information about neutrophil trafficking and kinetics [23]. The acute injury changes are distinct from the normal lung, PET-CT is used to evaluate this early inflammatory change. One of the hypotheses is FDG distribution volume increased with infiltrating neutrophils and phosphorylation rate with the regional expression of inflammatory cytokines such as IL-1 β, IL-8, and IL-10. Thus, the ARDS mechanism is based on the mechanism of injury with endotoxemia and surfactant depletion. Rodrigues et al. [24] studied patients with pulmonary contusion. He showed a diffuse uptake pattern of FDG after 1–3 days of blunt thoracic trauma with lung contusion.

In conclusion, PET-CT in ARDS shows quantitative pulmonary function and response to anti-inflammatory therapies which complementary to the existing conventional imaging modalities, which detect only anti-inflammatory changes.

14.6.3 Pulmonary Langerhans Cell Histiocytosis

Langerhans cell histiocytosis is a rare disease. The pathophysiology is associated with abnormal function of T-cell, macrophage, and/or cytokine-mediated process. The role of PET-CT here is to evaluate the base reactivity of inflammation involved in LCH, clinical assessment, and monitoring response to therapy [25, 26].

14.7   Abdomen

FDG PET-CT is also important to evaluate the various pathological entities. The various causes of infection and inflammatory pathologies in the pediatric age group are confined to major visceral organs like liver, spleen, kidneys, urinary bladder, urethra, peritoneum, bowel loops, and mesentery. Hepatitis, appendicitis, cholecystitis, pancreatitis, pyelonephritis, glomerulonephritis, cystitis, and inflammatory bowel diseases are important. All these conditions can be diagnosed by FDG PET-CT as a tracer focus in the respective region [27–30]. This has to be differentiated from various malignancies in various pediatric age groups (Fig. 14.6).

14.8   Fever in Immunocompromised Children

FDG PET-CT plays an important role in the evaluation of the fever in the cases of the immunocompromised children [6, 31]. Fever was defined as equal to or more than 38C, prolonged fever as fever more than or equal to 72 h, and recurrent fever as new fever after 48 hours of being afebrile with neutropenia. Bacteremia is defined as a recognized pathogen cultured from one or more blood cultures from two or more blood cultures drawn on two separate occasions. The role of FDG PET-CT is to have the potential to complement the various treatment regimes like antibacterial, antifungal, and others (Figs. 14.7, 14.8 and 14.9).

14.9   Limitations of PET-CT

The most important worry about some aspects of FDG PET-CT is radiation. ALARA principle has to be followed strictly in the evaluation of pediatric pathologies by FDG PET-CT [32, 33]. This is important to differentiate the various risks occurring

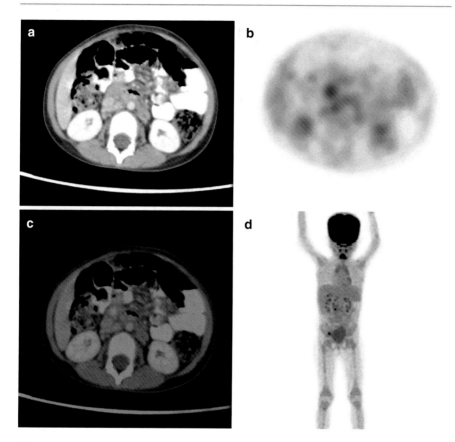

Fig. 14.6 Whole-body PET-CT CT image showing moderate right pleural effusion with collapse of the lung and nodular pleural thickening showing diffuse increased uptake with SUV max of 4.2. Bilateral uptake noted in epiphysis of shoulder, elbow, hip, knee, and ankle

because of radiation at various pediatric age groups and various organs. Before advising PET-CT for staging and for restaging, after the treatment has to be meticulously planned to keep in mind the radiation aspects. For this, PET-MRI has a little relief for the amount of radiation due to CT.

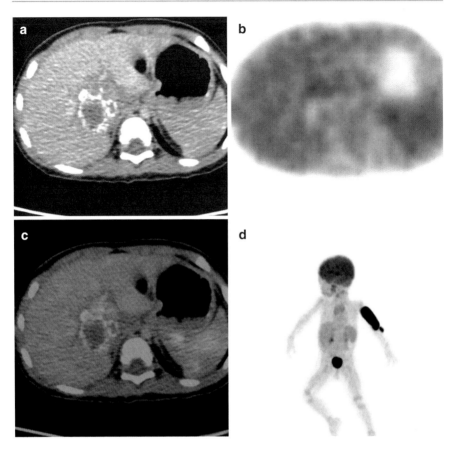

Fig. 14.7 CT image (**a**), small calcified lesion with no metabolic activity involving segment-I and V of the liver with no FDG uptake on PET images (**b**, **d**) a and fused images (**c**) suggestive of healed chronic organized abscess

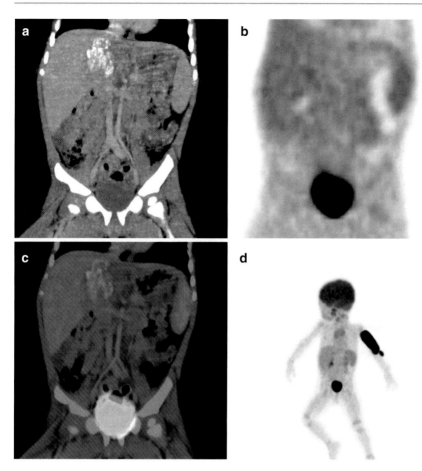

Fig. 14.8 CT image (**a**), small calcified lesion with no metabolic activity involving segment-I and V of the liver with no FDG uptake on PET images (**b**, **d**) and fused image (**c**) suggestive of healed chronic organized abscess

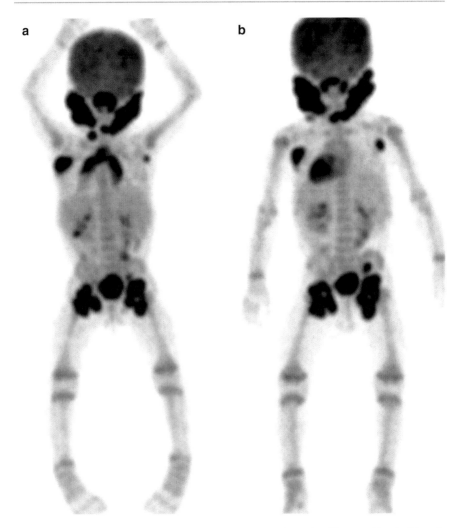

Fig. 14.9 PET images (**a**, **b**) showing diffuse cervical, mediastinal, axillary, and inguinal lymphadenopathy. Image (**a**) pre-therapy and Image (**b**) post-therapy in lymphoproliferative disorder

References

1. El-Radhi AS, Carroll J, Klein N. Clinical manual of fever in children. 1st ed. Berlin, Heidelberg: Springer; 2009.
2. Depas G, Decortis T, Francotte N, Bricteux G, Hustinx R. F-18 FDG PET in infectious diseases in children. Clin Nucl Med. 2011;8:593–8.
3. Servaes S. Imaging infection and inflammation in children with (18)F-FDG PET and (18) F-FDG PET/CT. J Nucl Med Technol. 2011;39(3):179–82.
4. del Rosal T, Goycochea WA, Mendez-Echevarria A, et al. ^{18}F-FDG PET/CT in the diagnosis of occult bacterial infections in children. Eur J Pediatr. 2013;172(8):1111–5.
5. Depas G, Decortis T, Francotte N, et al. F-18 FDG PET in infectious diseases in children. Clin Nucl Med. 2007;32(8):593–8.
6. Blokhuis GJ, Bleeker-Rovers CP, Diender MG, Oyen WJ, Draaisma JM, de Geus-Oei LF. Diagnostic value of FDG-PET/(CT) in children with fever of unknown origin and unexplained fever during immune suppression. Eur J Nucl Med Mol Imaging. 2014;41:1916–23.
7. Grant FD. Normal variations and benign findings in pediatric 18F-FDG-PET/CT. PET Clin. 2014;9(2):195–208.
8. Shammas A, Lim R, Charron M. Pediatric FDG PET/CT: physiologic uptake, normal variants, and benign conditions. Radiographics. 2009;29(5):1467–86.
9. Parisi MT, Otjen JP, Stanescu AL, et al. Radionuclide imaging of infection and inflammation in children: a review. Semin Nucl Med. 2018;48(2):148–65.
10. Chow A, Robinson JL. Fever of unknown origin in children: a systematic review. World J Pediatr. 2011;7(1):5–10.
11. Arora R, Mahajan P. Evaluation of child with fever without source: review of literature and update. Pediatr Clin N Am. 2013;60:1049–62. https://doi.org/10.1016/j.pcl.2013.06.009.
12. Abouzied MM, Crawford ES, Nabi HA. 18F-FDG imaging: pitfalls and artifacts. J Nucl Med Technol. 2005;33(3):145–55.
13. Burrell SC, Van den Abbeele AD. 2-Deoxy-2-[F-18] fluoro-D-glucose positron emission tomography of the head and neck: an atlas of normal uptake and variants. Mol Imaging Biol. 2005;7(3):244–56.
14. Vorster M, Maes A, de WCV, et al. Gallium-68PET: a powerful generator-based alternative to infection and inflammation imaging. Semin Nucl Med. 2016;46(5):436–47.
15. Kwon HW, Lee H-Y, Hwang Y-H, et al. Diagnostic performance of 18F-FDG-labeled white blood cell PET/CT for cyst infection in patients with autosomal dominant polycystic kidney disease: a prospective study. Nucl Med Commun. 2016 May;37(5):493–8.
16. Zhao Q, Dong A, Bai Y, et al. FDG PET/CT in immunoglobulin G4-related spinal hypertrophic pachymeningitis. Clin Nucl Med. 2017;42(12):958–61.
17. Gambhir S, Kumar M, Ravina M, et al. Role of [18] F-FDG PET in demonstrating disease burden in patients with tuberculous meningitis. J Neurol Sci. 2016 Nov 15;370:196–200.
18. Blodgett TM, Fukui MB, Snyderman CH, et al. Combined PET-CT in the head and neck: part 1. Physiologic, altered physiologic, and artifactual FDG uptake. Radiographics. 2005;25:897–912. https://doi.org/10.1148/rg.254035156.
19. Zhuang H, Yu JQ, Alavi A. Applications of fluorodeoxyglucose-PET imaging in the detection of infection and inflammation and other benign disorders. Radiol Clin N Am. 2005;43:121–34. https://doi.org/10.1016/j.rcl.2004.07.005.
20. Umeda Y, Demura Y, Ishizaki T, Ameshima S, Miyamori I, Saito Y, Tsuchida T, Fujibayashi Y, Okazawa H. Dual-time-point 18F-FDG PET imaging for diagnosis of disease type and disease activity in patients with idiopathic interstitial pneumonia. Eur J Nucl Med Mol Imaging 2009;36:1121–30.
21. Chen YM, Huang G, Sun XG, et al. Optimizing delayed scan time for FDG PET: comparison of the early and late delayed scan. Nucl Med Commun. 2008;29:425–30.
22. Amin R, Charron M, Grinblat L, et al. Cystic fibrosis: detecting changes in airway inflammation with FDG PET/CT. Radiology. 2012 Sep;264(3):868–75.

23. de Prost N, Tucci MR, Melo MFV, et al. Assessment of lung inflammation with ^{18}F-FDG PET during acute lung injury. AJR Am J Roentgenol. 2010 Aug;195(2):292–300.
24. Rodrigues RS, Miller PR, Bozza FA, Marchiori E, et al. FDG-PET in patients at risk for acute respiratory distress syndrome: a preliminary report. Intensive Care Med. 2008 Dec;34(12):2273–8.
25. Binkovitz LA, Olshefski RS, Adler BH. Coincidence FDG-PET in the evaluation of Langerhans' cell histiocytosis: preliminary findings. Pediatr Radiol. 2003;33(9):598 602.
26. Phillips M, Allen C, Gerson P, et al. Comparison of FDG-PET scans to conventional radiography and bone scans in management of Langerhans cell histiocytosis. Pediatr Blood Cancer. 2009;52(1):97–101.
27. Del Rosal T, Goycochea WA, Méndez-Echevarría A, García-Fernández de Villalta M, Baquero-Artigao F, Coronado M, et al. ^{18}F-FDG PET/CT in the diagnosis of occult bacterial infections in children. Eur J Pediatr. 2013;172(8):1111–5.
28. Tokmak H, Ergonul O, Demirkol O, Cetiner M, Ferhanoglu B. Diagnostic contribution of (18) F-FDG-PET/CT in fever of unknown origin. Int J Infect Dis. 2014;19:53–8.
29. Federici L, Blondet C, Imperiale A, et al. Value of (18)F-FDG-PET/CT in patients with fever of unknown origin and unexplained prolonged inflammatory syndrome: a single centre analysis experience. Int J Clin Pract. 2010;64:55–60.
30. Meller J, Sahlmann CO, Scheel AK. 18F-FDG PET and PET/CT in fever of unknown origin. J Nucl Med. 2007 Jan;48(1):35–45.
31. García-Gómez FJ, Acevedo-Báñez I, Martínez-Castillo R, et al. Usefulness of (18)FDG PET-CT scan as a diagnostic tool of fever of unknown origin. Med Clin (Barc). 2015 Jul 20;145(2):62–6.
32. Chawla SC, Federman N, Zhang D, et al. Estimated cumulative radiation dose from PET/CT in children with malignancies: a 5-year retrospective review. Pediatr Radiol. 2010;40:681–6.
33. Gelfand MJ, Lemen LC. PET/CT and SPECT/CT dosimetry in children: the challenge to the pediatric imager. Semin Nucl Med. 2007;37:391–8.

PET-CT in Musculoskeletal Infection and Inflammation

15

Key Points

With the evolution of technology and radiotracers, PET-CT has become an important imaging modality to evaluate the infection and inflammatory process. FDG is the most commonly used radiotracer; however, newer radiotracers are also under preclinical research.

The biggest advantage is noninvasive whole-body evaluation in a single scan. Common radiotracers used for different pathologies like FDG, 18F NaF, Gallium 68 are used for various applications. Various pathologies involving muscles, nerves, skeletons, and joints can be evaluated. Recently PET-MR is going to be a very crucial imaging modality for final details of cartilage, synovium, muscles, and neurovascular bundles.

15.1 Introduction

Molecular imaging in the musculoskeletal system has evolved with the advent of hybrid imaging modalities like PET-CT, SPECT-CT, and PET-MR. These imaging modalities give valuable information related to the molecular and cell biology of the musculoskeletal system. Conventional imaging modalities are usually used for the diagnosis of various pathologies in the musculoskeletal system. These modalities show anatomical changes which can be seen in a late phase in these modalities. However, PET-CT being the molecular imaging modality shows the pathological changes very early at the onset of the disease [1–3].

15.2   PET-CT Imaging

15.2.1 FDG

FDG glucose is the most widely used radiotracer for metabolism and can be easily distinguished by the PET scan. The biochemical process is via glucose transporters, which have an affinity for infection and inflammation. FDG is transported easily into the perfused areas which accumulate in any pathological area in acute or chronic stage of the infection [4].

15.2.2 18F NaF PET-CT Scan

Bone tissue is undergoing rapid remodeling every time. F-18 exchanged on the surface of hydroxyapatite to form fluorapatite thus the uptake on PET images is based on osteolytic and osteoblastic processes. NaF scan is extremely sensitive for evaluating the remodeling of the bone secondary to infection and inflammation [5] (Fig. 15.1).

15.2.3 18F Fluorodeoxyglucose Labelled Leukocyte Scan

This leukocyte scan is important for specific imaging of infection where leukocytes are labeled with F-18 FDG. The basis of this scan is leukocyte accumulation at the site of inflammation [6]. This forms the basis of the uptake depending on the leucocyte metabolism in the various infections.

15.2.4 Ga-68-Citrate PET-CT Scan

Ga-68-Citrate scan is sensitive for inflammation, trauma, and tumor. The shorter half-life of Ga-68 is an advantage for these scans [7].

15.3   Various Indications of PET-CT in Musculoskeletal System

15.3.1 Osteomyelitis

Osteomyelitis is an acute or chronic inflammatory disease involving the bone marrow and adjacent bone secondary to pyogenic organisms. It is classified into several types depending on the patient's age, onset of disease, root of infection, and etiology. The predisposing factors for osteomyelitis are diabetes mellitus, AIDS, IV drug abuse, alcoholism, chronic steroid use, immunosuppression, chronic joint disease, any surgeries, fractures, and orthopedic implants or devices [8, 9]. The types of

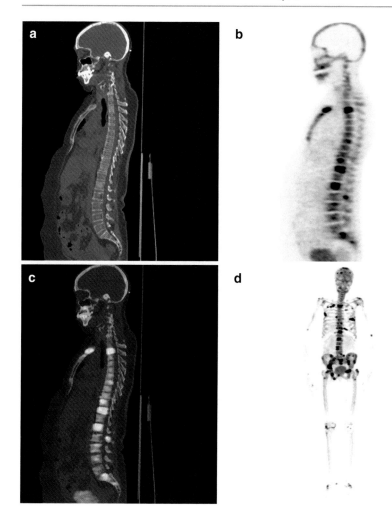

Fig. 15.1 F-18 bone scan showing multiple vertebral body sclerosis on CT image (**a**) with significant uptake on PET images (**b**) and (**d**) and fused image (**c**) suggestive of metastases

osteomyelitis are acute hematogenous osteomyelitis, osteitis, chronic osteomyelitis, acute on chronic osteomyelitis, osteomyelitis with associated pathological conditions like a diabetic foot. FDG PET-CT shows the metabolic activity corresponding to the disease activity in the associated bones. Zhuang and colleagues [10] investigated 22 patients with possible chronic osteomyelitis and the FDG PET findings whereas follows sensitivity, specificity, and accuracy of 100%, 87.5%, and 91%, respectively. Meller co-workers [11] published a prospective analysis of 29 patients for possible chronic osteomyelitis. The FDG PET-CT showed a sensitivity of 100% and specificity of 95%.

Osteomyelitis is one of the commonest infections involving the skeletal system. FDG PET-CT has become the most important imaging modality with sensitivity and specificity of more than 90% in most of the studies [12]. FDG PET-CT is equally sensitive in postoperative settings where inflammation persists for 4–6 weeks post-operatively. FDG PET-CT is equally important in the evaluation of chronic osteomyelitis are presenting with the symptoms of osteomyelitis for more than 6 weeks. PET-CT plays a similar role in the evaluation and monitoring of therapy response in patients with osteomyelitis. In one of the studies done in the pediatric age group by Warmann and colleagues [13], FDG PET is highly sensitive in differentiating between infection and reparative activity within the musculoskeletal system after treatment of acute osteomyelitis. These FDG findings are consistent with various laboratory findings and clinical status in both evaluation and follow up after therapy.

15.3.2 Infective Spondylodiscitis

Spondylodiscitis is a common entity in relation to the fever of unknown origin where bacteremia is an important component. FDG PET-CT plays an important role in the evaluation of infection, associated degenerative changes, and infection. PET-CT has the advantage to reduce the artifacts secondary to metallic implants, plate, and screws or stabilization devices. In all these conditions, PET has an advantage compared to other conventional imaging modalities which have limited results. PET-CT is important for discriminating degenerative changes from the discitis where it can be quantified by the amount of FDG uptake [14]. There are a lot of false-positive findings secondary to associated findings like tumor, focal inflammation, and early degenerative changes (Figs. 15.2, 15.3, 15.4 and 15.5).

15.3.3 Diabetic Foot

Diabetic foot is one of the important complications of diabetes caused by the involvement of peripheral vascular disease and neuropathy or a combination of both. Charcot arthropathy is one of the important entities in relation to diabetes where noninfectious soft tissue inflammation with destruction of joints and bones. FDG PET-CT has become an important imaging modality in imaging bone infection and associated soft tissue involvement in a form of diabetic foot and cellulitis. A study done by Nawaz and colleagues [15] showed significant promising results with sensitivity, specificity, positive predictive value (PPV), negative predictive value (NPV), and accuracy of 81%, 93%, 78%, 94%, and 90%, respectively. PET-CT plays an important role to differentiate between osteomyelitis and Charcot's arthropathy. Hopfner and colleagues [16] studied the role of FDG PET for pre-operative identification of neuropathy joints in patients with diabetes. Significant high SUV max was noted in this and thus FDG PET-CT could differentiate between

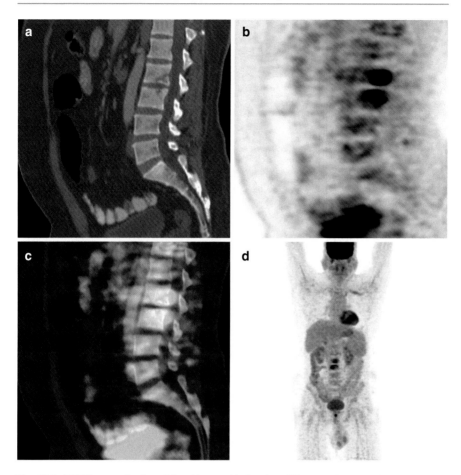

Fig. 15.2 PET images (**b**, **d**) and fused image (**c**) showing diffuse uptake along the endplates of L2-L3 with erosion seen on CT image (**a**) suggestive of infective spondylodiscitis

osteomyelitis and neuropathic disease. FDG PET had differentiated between osteomyelitis and Charcot's by the amount of uptake.

15.3.4 Prosthetic Joint Infections

PET-CT has an important role in the evaluation of prosthetic joints between loosening and infection after surgery. Lawrence and Yogurt et al. [17] reported 100% sensitivity and 73% specificity for prosthetic knee infections. Basu and colleagues [18] found the PET-CT was more specific and sensitive for prosthetic hip infections. In a recent meta-analysis, the pooled sensitivity and specificity of 18F FDG PET and PET-CT for lower extremity prosthetic joint infection both were 86%.

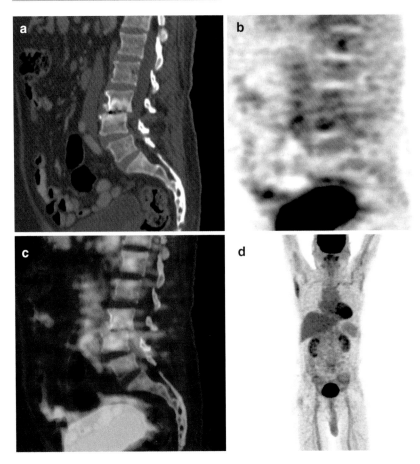

Fig. 15.3 PET images (**b, d**) and fused image (**c**) showing diffuse uptake along the endplates of L2-L3 with erosion and endplate sclerosis on CT image (**a**) suggestive of infective spondylodiscitis

15.3.5 Collagen Disorders

Various collagen disorders like Polymyalgia Rheumatic, SLE (Systemic Lupus Erythematosus), Seronegative spondyloarthropathies, psoriatic arthritis, ankylosing spondylitis, and other idiopathic inflammatory arthropathies. FDG is a promising modality for the clinical assessment of these conditions. FDG PET delineates the inflammatory activity along with the articular and extraarticular sites, which can be correlated with the clinical symptoms. The uptake in these joints is directly proportional to the amount of disease activity in these regions. Diffuse increased uptake also noted along the tendons enthuses and in the name bed in various conditions, especially psoriatic arthritis that correlates with tenosynovitis, enthesitis, and nail dystrophy [19]. FDG PET-CT also has a significant role in adult-onset still disease,

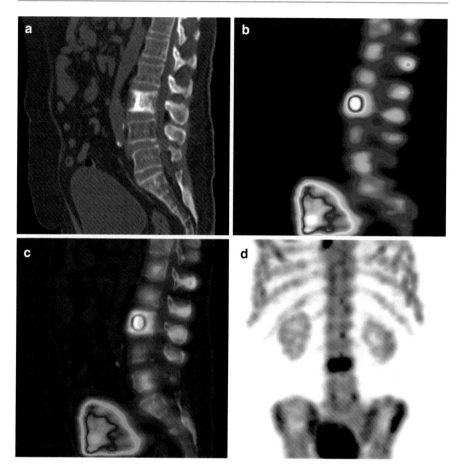

Fig. 15.4 CT image (**a**) showing diffuse L3 vertebral sclerosis with significant uptake on SPECT-CT images (**b, c, d**) and associated anterior aspect erosion on suggestive of infective inflammatory

hemophagocytic lymphohistiocytosis showing significant hypermetabolism in the notes, bone marrow, spleen, and multiple joints which are involved.

15.3.6 Osteonecrosis

FDG PET and 18F NaF PET also plays an important role in the evaluation of osteo-necrosis of the bone in the affected patients. These radiotracers show increased focal uptake which is corresponding with the severity of osteonecrosis [20]. The avascular necrosis involving bones, especially femoral heads also show increased FDG activity and hypermetabolism which is corresponding with the disease activity.

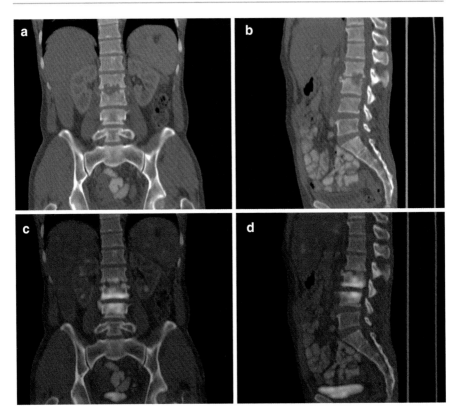

Fig. 15.5 PET-CT fused images (**c**, **d**) images showing diffuse uptake along the endplates of L2-L3 with erosion and endplate sclerosis seen on CT images (**a**, **b**) suggestive of infective spondylodiscitis

15.3.7 Osteoporosis

18 NaF PET shows a significant role in the evaluation of osteoporosis, which can quantify the regional or site-specific bone changes. SUV measurements are usually lower in the osteoporotic bones compared to healthy patients and correspond with bone mineral density [21] (Figs. 15.6 and 15.7).

15.4   Evaluation of Inflammatory Vasculopathies Affecting Muscles

FDG PET-CT is establishing a major role in the evaluation of various inflammatory vasculopathies in conditions of large vessel vasculitis, medium vessel vasculitis, Takayasu's arteritis, joint cell arteritis, aortitis, SLE, Polyarteritis Nodosa, and Churg-Strauss syndrome. The changes in the muscles in relation to the involvement of the muscle and uptake corresponds to the severity of the disease [22].

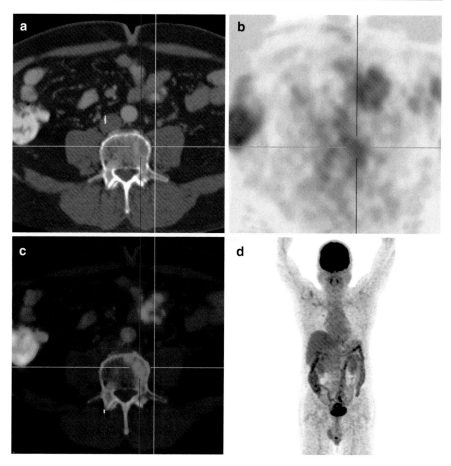

Fig. 15.6 Whole-body PET-CT at the level of L4 vertebral body showing small subtle lytic area in left side of vertebral body on CT image (**a**) with minimal uptake on PET images (**b, d**) and fused image (**c**) with SUV max of 2.5

15.5   Evaluation of Fractures and Complications

Evaluation of fractures is one of the important incidental findings during routine workup of whole-body PET-CT scans. These fractures can be traumatic, surgical, or pathological fractures. The amount of FDG corresponds with this fracture site and depends on the acuteness of the fracture. The acute fracture more the FDG uptake. In the pathological malignant settings, they play an important role in the differentiation from the metastatic focus vs. pathological fracture vs. traumatic. The quantification is done by SUV max values less than 2.4 benign and more than 2.4 are supposed to be malignant. FDG PET also plays significant role in the evaluation of fracture non-union or any other associated obligations. The non-union has to be

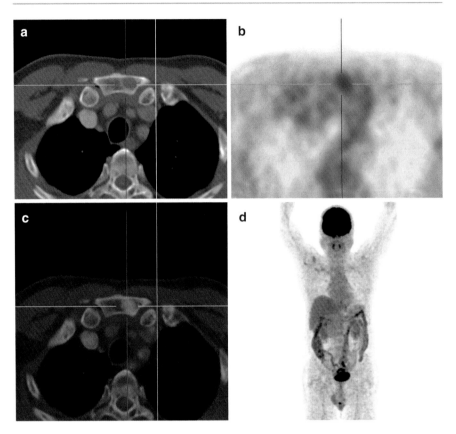

Fig. 15.7 Whole-body PET-CT at the level of sternum showing small subtle lytic area on CT image (**a**) and with minimal uptake on PET images (**b**) and (**d**) and fused image (**c**) with SUV max of 2.8

differentiated from associated or superadded infection. In patients with equivocal clinical findings, the sensitivity, specificity, positive predictive value, negative predictive value, and accuracy of FDG PET-CT for the evaluation of infected nonunited fractures are 85%, 86%, 79%, 90%, and 86%, respectively [23]. 18F NaF PET has an in vivo indicator of osteoblastic activity can detect fracture non-union at an early time point and play an important role in monitoring of healing fractures [24] (Figs. 15.8 and 15.9).

15.6   Inflammatory Osteoarthropathies

Inflammatory osteoarthropathies are a diverse group of autoimmune disorders, which have varying clinical features and prognosis. PET-CT plays an important role in the assessment of joint inflammation [25] for diagnostic assessment and to evaluate the monitoring response to therapy.

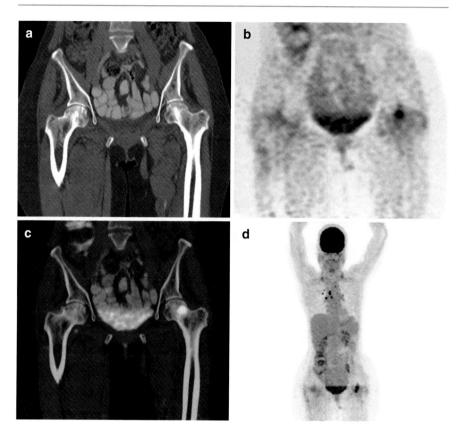

Fig. 15.8 Whole-body PET-CT with images at hip joint showing diffuse increased uptake at the left femoral neck images (**b, c, d**) associated with subtle lucency in CT image (**a**) with SUV max of 4.9 suggestive of impacted left femoral neck fracture

15.7   Miscellaneous

FDG PET-CT is evolving as an important imaging modality for the various incidental or miscellaneous conditions like metabolic bone disorders. Posttreatment evaluation of various conditions and few benign conditions which can be associated with infection. The concept theory is increased FDG uptake corresponding to the disease activity. But the underlying clinical setting has to be kept in mind, for example, diffuse marrow uptake in an adult can be reactive, can be metabolic change, can be secondary to some treatment changes, or can be disseminated infective inflammatory changes.

15.8   Septic Arthritis

Septic arthritis is a component of infectious arthritis, which has direct, hematogenous spread, or contiguous spread from an adjacent intraarticular site of infection. Conventional imaging modalities like ultrasound and MRI and bone scan are not

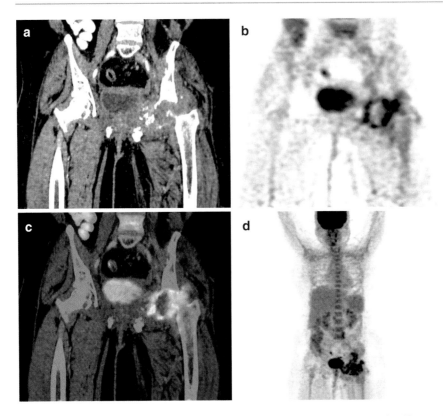

Fig. 15.9 Whole-body PET-CT at the level of hip joints CT image A showing ill-defined large soft tissue component with the destruction of bones of hip joint and displacement image (**a**). This soft tissue shows significant uptake on PET images (**b, d**) and fused image (**c**) with SUV max of 5.8. No history of trauma, but a long history of hip pain and fever on and off for the last 7 months. The findings are suggestive of extensive infective arthritis

considered as sensitive modalities. FDG PET role in septic arthritis is limited. However, newer radiotracers like Gallium and labeled leukocytes are more specific and with them the role of PET is more promising [26].

15.9 Rheumatoid Arthritis

Rheumatoid arthritis is an autoimmune disease involving the systemic joints with acute and chronic inflammation of the joints. The pathophysiology results in synovitis and pannus formation resulting in increased FDG uptake. A lot of studies have evaluated the role of FDG PET in patients with rheumatoid arthritis [27]. The amount of the FDG uptake in affected joints correlates with the clinical symptoms, disease activity, swelling, tenderness, and associated constitutional symptoms. There is neovascularization of the synovium, which shows increased uptake. FDG

PET has a higher sensitivity than clinical symptoms. FDG PET has an important role in assessing the treatment response to antirheumatic drug therapy in patients with rheumatoid arthritis [28]. FDG PET plays an important role in the evaluation of other joint pathologies if one or two joints are involved.

15.10 Psoriasis

Psoriasis is an inflammatory condition involving the skin and causing psoriatic arthritis. FDG PET has a great potential to visualize the extent and ability of psoriatic arthritis. FDG PET shows the arthritic involvement of joints and enthuses in asymptomatic psoriasis. It is also important to evaluate the treatment response with tumor necrosis factor a (TNF-a) [29].

15.11 Osteoarthritis

Osteoarthritis is a degenerative joint disease involving the cartilage with cartilaginous degradation, subchondral bony sclerosis, and osteophyte formation. This osteoarthritis involves multiple joints, commonest is the knee joint because of weight-bearing property and continuous wear and tear.

Osteoarthritis is the commonest form of arthritis worldwide. The commonest joints involved are hip and knee joints. Osteoarthritis is characterized by loss of articular cartilage and remodeling of the underlying bone. Nakamura and colleagues [30] showed that the amount of FDG uptake periarticular lesions than articular cartilage varies with the stage of osteoarthritis. PET-CT also is an important diagnostic tool to detect joint inflammation and assessing the severity of the disease. 18F NaF PET scan plays an important role in accessing the metabolic activity of changes in cartilage and bone remodeling [31]. NaF plays an important role in evaluating degenerative and arthritic joints earlier than the routine conventional imaging modalities. Other conditions like synovitis, hyperostosis, osteitis syndrome, psoriatic arthritis, collagen vascular disease-associated arthritis, juvenile idiopathic arthritis, ankylosing spondylitis, reactive arthritis can be evalauted by NaF. One of the important advantages for the PET-CT compared to other imaging modalities is the evalaution of SUV values which can signifies the early changes compared to other modalities, especially when the symptoms are mild. Another application for PET-CT is to localize the painful abnormalities in the inflamed joints and to differentiate between moderate and severe osteoarthritis. In the early phase these conditions can be made reversible by the available general and individualized therapies. The commonest form of lifestyle changes like weight loss and exercise as well as medications like NSAIDs, Acetaminophen, and Tramadol as per ACR guidelines. One of the important implications for PET to guide the targeted therapy in the joint for relief of osteoarthritic changes. However, this is not widely used. FDG PET is effectively used for quantifying the inflammatory activity of arthritis and response to treatment.

15.12 18F Fluoride Bone Scan

18F fluoride bone scan also plays an important role in the evaluation of osteoarthritis. This is again consistent with the amount of uptake that is directly proportional to the amount of degenerative changes. A lot of other pathologies like associated bone marrow changes, posttraumatic, metabolic bone disease, and malignant pathologies have to be ruled out [32, 33].

15.13 Myositis

Myositis is an inflammatory disorder involving the muscles clinically presented as muscle weakness and fatigue. This can be associated with malignancies and paraneoplastic syndromes. The role of PET depends on the amount of inflammation or infection involving the particular muscles. The biggest disadvantage is physical exercise or any movement after injecting the FDG which will give the muscle scan. FDG PET is important in evaluating the metabolic activity in traumatic myopathies, infections, and diabetic muscle infarction, rhabdomyolysis, and after physical exercise [34, 35]. The FDG PET is an important imaging modality to provide the various range of information (Figs. 15.10 and 15.11).

Cutaneous lesions or nodules also show focal FDG uptake (Fig. 15.12).

15.14 Imaging of Pain

Pain is an important and most common medical attention by the patients. It can be acute or chronic and the diagnosis and characterization of pain are challenging. Clinical assessment is subjective to the patient's response. Structural imaging modalities are not much of relevance. Due to this, FDG PET plays an important role to identify the neural activity to localize the pain if any nerve involvement is there [36]. This is not sensitive, but many studies are going on. In one of the studies where patient presented with progressive difficulty in walking there was increased FDG focus seen in lower spinal cord and sciatic nerves consistent with signs of neuropathy [37]. The role of PET-MR is more crucial because of high sensitivity assessment of affected nerves. FDG PET-CT has evolved as a promising tool in assisting various infective and inflammatory processes in the musculoskeletal system. It has very high sensitivity specificity, noninvasive, less time-consuming when tolerated by patients in a single whole-body imaging protocol. Various radiotracers as described above are used for infection inflammation but along with these newer radiotracers are being explored for the same. PET-MR is having an added value for minor details of cartilage muscles and nerves.

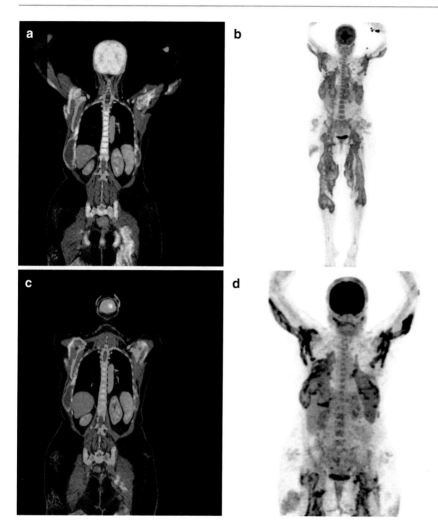

Fig. 15.10 Whole-body PET-CT, PET images (**b**, **d**), and fused images (**a**, **d**) showing diffuse uptake along the muscles secondary to collections in all the muscles with significant FDG uptake. This FDG uptake shows SUV max of 5.5 suggestive of myositis collections

Newer radiotracers like DOTONAC [38] and PSMA [39] which are used for neuroendocrine tumors and prosthetic tumors also show bone pathologies like osteoarthritis, benign bony lesions, and metastatic bone lesions.

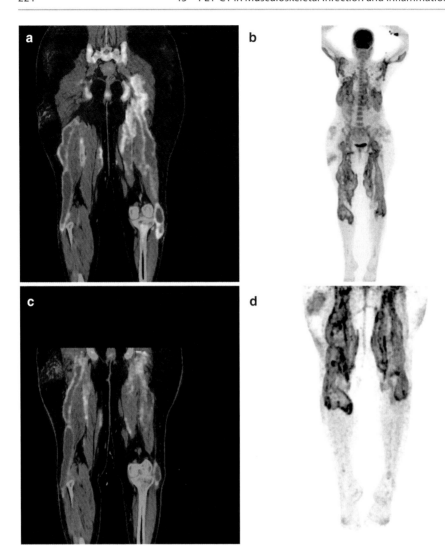

Fig. 15.11 Whole-body PET-CT, PET images (**b**, **d**), and fused image (**a**, **c**) showing diffuse uptake along the muscles secondary to collections in all the muscles with significant FDG uptake. This FDG uptake shows SUV max of 5.5 suggestive of myositis collections

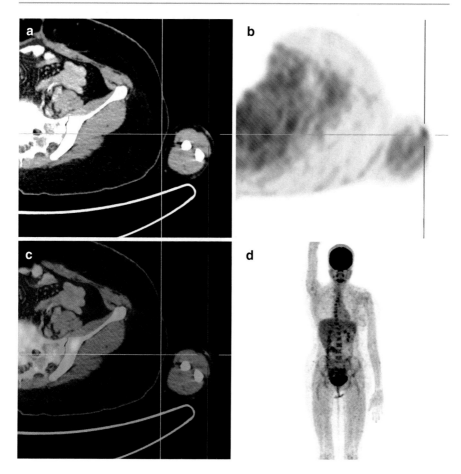

Fig. 15.12 Whole-body PET-CT at the level of left forearm showing tiny nodular lesion in the subcutaneous plane and skin on CT image (**a**) with mild FDG uptake on PET images (**b, d**) and fused images (**c**) with SUV max of 3.9 suggestive of cutaneous inflammatory nodule

15.15 Conclusion

Thus, PET plays a significant role in the evaluation of musculoskeletal infective and inflammatory pathologies by using radiotracers like FDG, 18 NaF, DOTONAC, and PSMA.

References

1. Osman DR. Diagnosis and management of musculoskeletal infection. In: Fitzgerald RH, Haufer H, Malkani RL, editors. Orthopedics. St. Louis: Mosby; 2002. p. 695–707.

2. Love C, Tomas MB, Tronco GG, et al. Imaging infection and inflammation with 18F-FDG-PET. Radiographics. 2005;25:1357–68.
3. Strobel K, KDM S. PET/CT in musculoskeletal infection. Semin Musculoskelet Radiol. 2007;11:353–64.
4. Kalicke T, Schmitz A, Risse JH, et al. Fluorine-18 fluorodeoxyglucose PET in infectious bone diseases: results of histologically confirmed cases. Eur J Nucl Med Mol Imaging. 2000;27:524–8.
5. Apolo AB, Lindenberg L, Shih JH, Mena E, Kim JW, Park JC, et al. Prospective study evaluating Na18F PET/CT in predicting clinical outcomes and survival in advanced prostate cancer. J Nucl Med. 2016;57(6):886–92.
6. Yilmaz S, Aliyev A, Ekmekcioglu O, Ozhan M, Uslu L, Vatankulu B, Sager S, Halaç M, Sönmezoğlu K. Comparison of FDG and FDG-labeled leukocytes PET/CT in diagnosis of infection. Nuklearmedizin. 2015;54:262–71.
7. Salomaki SP, Kemppainen J, Hohenthal U, et al. Head-to-head comparison of (68)Ga-citrate and (18)F-FDG PET/CT for detection of infectious foci in patients with *Staphylococcus aureus* Bacteraemia. Contrast Media Mol Imaging. 2017;2017:3179607.
8. Makis W, Stern J. Chronic vascular graft infection with fistula to bone causing vertebral osteomyelitis, imaged with F-18 FDG PET/CT. Clin Nucl Med. 2010;35(10):794–6.
9. Guhlmann A, Brecht-Krauss D, Suger G, et al. Fluorine-18-FDG PET and technetium-99 mantigranulocyte antibody scintigraphy in chronic osteomyelitis. J Nucl Med. 1998;39:2145–52.
10. Zhuang H, Duarte PS, Pourdehand M, et al. Exclusion of chronic osteomyelitis with F-18 fluorodeoxyglucose positron emission tomographic imaging. Clin Nucl Med. 2000;25:281–4.
11. Meller J, Koster G, Liersch T, et al. Chronic bacterial osteomyelitis: prospective comparison of F-18-FDG imaging with a dual-head coincidence camera and In-111-labelled autologousleucocyte scintigraphy. Eur J Nucl Med Mol Imaging. 2002;29:53–60.
12. Nakamura H, Masuko K, Yudoh K, et al. Positron emission tomography with ^{18}F-FDG in osteoarthritic knee. Osteoarthr Cartil. 2007;15(6):673–81.
13. Warmann SW, Dittmann H. Guido Seitz follow-up of acute osteomyelitis in children: the possible role of PET/CT in selected cases. J Pediatr Surg. 2011;46(8):1550–6.
14. Schmitz A, Risse JH, Grunwald F, et al. Fluorine-18 fluorodeoxyglucose positron emission tomography findings in spondylodiscitis: preliminary results. Eur Spine J. 2001;10:534–9.
15. Nawaz A, Torigian DA, Siegelman ES, et al. Diagnostic performance of FDG-PET, MRI, and plain film radiography(PFR) forth diagnosis of osteomyelitis in the diabetic foot. Mol Imaging Biol. 2010;12:335–42.
16. Hopfner S, Krolak C, Kessler S, et al. Pre-operative imaging of Charcot neuroarthropathy in diabetic patients: comparison of ring PET, hybrid PET, and magnetic resonance imaging. Foot Ankle Int. 2004;25:890–5.
17. Lawrence E., et al. Periprosthetic joint infections: clinical and bench research. Sci World J. 2013. 549091, 17 p.
18. Basu S, Kwee TC, Hess S. FDG-PET/CT imaging of infected bones and prosthetic joints. Curr Mol Imaging. 2014;3(3):225–9.
19. Suto T, Okamura K, Yonemoto Y, Okura C, Tsushima Y, Takagishi K. Prediction of large joint destruction in patients with rheumatoid arthritis using 18F-FDG PET/CT and disease activity score. Medicine (Baltimore). 2016;95:e2841.
20. Alhilali L, Reynolds AR, Fakhran S. Osteoradionecrosis after radiation therapy for head and neck cancer. differentiation from recurrent disease with CT and PET/CT imaging. AJNR Am J Neuroradiol. 2014;35:1405–11. https://doi.org/10.3174/ajnr.A3879.
21. Katzel JA, Heiba SI. PET/CT F-18 FDG scan accurately identifies osteoporotic fractures in a patient with known metastatic colorectal cancer. Clin Nucl Med. 2005;30(10):651–4.
22. Loffler C, Hoffend J, Benck U, Kramer BK, Bergner R. The value of ultrasound in diagnosing extracranial large-vessel vasculitis compared to FDG-PET/CT: a retrospective study. Clin Rheumatol. 2017;36:2079.
23. Shon IH, Fogelman I. F-18 FDG positron emission tomography and benign fractures. Clin Nucl Med. 2003;28(3):171–5.

24. Jadvar H, Desai B, Conti PS. Sodium 18 F-fluoride PET/CT of bone, joint, and other disorders. Semin Nucl Med. 2015;1:58–65. https://doi.org/10.1053/j.semnuclmed.2014.07.008.
25. Yamada S, Kubota K, Kubota R, Ido T, Tamahashi N. High accumulation of fluorine-18-fluorodeoxyglucose in turpentine-induced inflammatory tissue. J Nucl Med. 1995;36:1301–6.
26. Stumpe KD, Notzli HP, Zanetti M, et al. FDG PET for differentiation of infection and aseptic loosening into total hip replacements: comparison with conventional radiography and three-phase bone scintigraphy. Radiology. 2004;231:333–41.
27. Rheumatoid arthritis. The intense FDG accumulation in both hip joints can be noted. As with single photon emitting tracers, it is not likely that FDG plays a significant role in the diagnosis of the septic joint. FDG-PET in musculoskeletal infections 375 associated infections with FDG PET in patients with trauma: correlation with microbiologic results. Radiology. 2003;226:391–8.
28. Beckers C, Ribbens C, Andre B, Marcelis S, Kaye O, Mathy L, et al. Assessment of disease activity in rheumatoid arthritis with (18)F-FDG PET. J Nucl Med. 2004;45:956–64.
29. Mehta NN, Yu YD, Saboury B. Systemic and vascular inflammation in patients with moderate to severe psoriasis as measured by [18F]-fluorodeoxyglucose positron emission tomography/computed tomography (FDG-PET/CT): a pilot study. Arch Dermatol. 2011;147(9):1031–9.
30. Kamekura S, Hoshi K, Nakamura K, et al. Osteoarthritis development in novel experimental mouse models induced by knee joint instability. Osteoarthr Cartil. 2005;13(7):632–41.
31. Fischer DR. Musculoskeletal imaging using fluoride PET. Semin Nucl Med. 2013;43:427–33.
32. Even-Sapir E, Mishani E, Flusser G, Metser U. 18F-fluoride positron emission tomography and positron emission tomography/computed tomography. Semin Nucl Med. 2007;37:462–9.
33. Wong KK, Piert M. Dynamic bone imaging with 99mTc-labeled diphosphonates and 18FNaF: mechanisms and applications. J Nucl Med. 2013;54:590–9.
34. Pipitone N, Versari A, Zuccoli G, et al. ^{18}F-fluorodeoxyglucose positron emission tomography for the assessment of myositis: a case series. Clin Exp Rheumatol. 2012;30:570–3.
35. hrapko BE, Chrapko M, Nocun A, Stefaniak B, Zubilewicz T, Drop A. Role of 18F-FDG PET/CT in the diagnosis of inflammatory and infectious vascular disease. Nucl Med Rev Cent East Eur. 2016;19:28–36. https://doi.org/10.5603/NMR.2016.0006.
36. Even-Sapir E, Metser U, Mishani E, Lievshitz G, Lerman H, Leibovitch I. The detection of bone metastases in patients with high-risk prostate cancer: 99mTc-MDP planar bone scintigraphy, single- and multi-field-of-view SPECT, 18F-fluoride PET, and 18F-fluoride PET/CT. J Nucl Med. 2006;47(2):287–97.
37. Cheng G, Chamroonrat W, Bing Z, et al. Elevated FDG activity in the spinal cord and the sciatic nerves due to neuropathy. Clin Nucl Med. 2009;34(12):950–1.
38. Kuyumcu S, Özkan ZG, Sanli Y, et al. Physiological and tumoral uptake of (68) Ga-DOTATATE: standardized uptake values and challenges in interpretation. Ann Nucl Med. 2013;27:538–45. https://doi.org/10.1007/s12149-013-0718-4.
39. Pomykala KL, Czernin J, Tristan R. Grogan total-body [68] Ga-PSMA-11 PET/CT for bone metastasis detection in prostate cancer patients: potential impact on bone scan guidelines. J Nucl Med. 2020;61(3):405–11.

PET-CT in Evaluation of Prosthetic Joint Infections

16

Key Points

Prosthetic joint infection is one of the less common infections which is detected due to advancements in the technology related to the imaging modalities and protocols. The most important thing is to differentiate between joint infection and aseptic loosening of the prosthesis. Postsurgical evaluation of the prosthesis is particularly important. Routine conventional modalities are not much sensitive for the evaluation and most of the time they are of not much use. Because of this, the infection and the cause cannot be ascertained. FDG PET-CT is widely used in oncology and the various associated and incidental finding's detection in oncological set-up now is now being used for various pathology evalautions and joint prosthesis evaluation is one of them. The other radiotracers used are related with the affinity of the infective focus detection like Indium leukocyte scan and 99tc sulfur colloid scan. The same principle is being used for the evaluation. FDG is mostly used and another reason is the very high sensitivity for the periprosthetic soft tissue uptake as well.

16.1 Introduction

Arthritis of the joints is common in older age groups, and the important reason is the loss of calcium due to various causes and other predisposing factors. Surgical field is also growing with the technology, and with the easily available newer techniques, a number of joint surgeries are planned and the success rate is quite high. Surgery is mostly done for degenerative arthritis rather than other causes of arthritis. After the surgery, most of the cases do not develop any complications but still a few cases can be varying from mild to severe form leading to rejection. For this type of cases, no clear guidelines are placed to evaluate them systematically. With this, the approach to evaluation is hampered. Musculoskeletal Infection Society and International Consensus Meeting are widely used in the diagnosis of PJI. The hip and knee joint

© The Author(s), under exclusive license to Springer Nature
Singapore Pte Ltd. 2021
S. Shaikh, *PET-CT in Infection and Inflammation*,
https://doi.org/10.1007/978-981-15-9801-2_16

prosthesis implantation can significantly improve the quality of life with associated arthritis [1, 2].

16.2   Various Imaging Modalities

The variable imaging modalities are not sensitive to pick up the early metabolic changes. The imaging modalities depend on the center-to-center availability, protocols set, and depending on the experience and equipment. By the time this can be picked up in the conventional modalities, the morbidity will be significantly on the higher side. So, this needs to be of concern. For this, the PET-CT is the modality of choice as a whole-body examination can be done in 1 h and any other focus of infection can be evaluated at the same time. Thus, PET-CT is being used to determine the early changes and the findings which cannot be picked up by routine imaging. Various laboratory investigations along with the imaging will help for better sensitivity. The various aspects which need to be diagnosed in the joint replacements are any aseptic loosening, fracture, and dislocation [3–5].

16.3   Clinical Diagnosis

Postsurgical infections are common in many surgical conditions and this joint prosthesis also is important. This identification is based on various clinical symptoms, various laboratory parameters, and if necessary, histopathological evaluation. The common clinical findings are pain, fever, inflammation, discharge, delayed healing and wound dehiscence, fistula from the joint, abscess, collection and necrosis, functional joint disorders in the form of stiffness, and reduced range of mobility. The most important clinical presentation is pain. Fever is nonspecific. Other predisposing factors are coagulopathy, diabetes, hypertension, previous surgeries, etc. The evacuation of the joint is based on the infection to identify the focus, associated periosteal reaction, osteolysis, calcifications, sinus tract description, extent of infection, joint space, stability of the joint, stability of the prosthesis, and soft tissue involvement. These are the major areas where the most of the modalities are not able to answer. So, in future, the role of these newer imaging modalities needs to be more concrete.

16.4   Differentiation of Periprosthetic Joint Infection

This evaluation by FDG PET is mostly based on major or minor criteria.

Primary Outcome
The diagnostic outcome of PJI with the minor criteria of the 2018 new definition (before and after revision).

Secondary Outcomes

The following will be assessed:

- Sensitivity, specificity, true-negative, false-positive, false-positive, positive predictive value, and negative predictive value (before and after revision)
- Sensitivity, specificity, true-negative, false-positive, false-positive, positive predictive value, and negative predictive value of the MSIS criteria.
- Sensitivity, specificity, true-negative, false-positive, false-positive, positive predictive value, and negative predictive value ICM Criteria
- Sensitivity, specificity, true-negative, false-positive, false-positive, positive predictive value, and negative predictive value IDSA Criteria.

This is based on the laboratory findings and complete detailed patient history and presentation and various tests. These various tests are in relation to serum, synovium, and postoperative. Serum indicators are C-reactive protein (CRP), D-dimer, interleukin-6 (IL-6), and erythrocyte sedimentation rate (ESR). Synovial indicators are white blood cells, leukocyte esterase, synovial alpha defensin, synovial polymorphonuclear neutrophil percentage (PMN), and synovial CRP. Intraoperative indicators are patient clinical data and any cultures. With this, the final outcome will decide the sensitivity, specificity, true-positive, true-negative, false-positive, false-negative, positive predictive value, and negative predictive value.

16.4.1 Inclusion Criteria

1. The patients fulfilling the major criteria like who are having sinus tract communication with the joint are two positive cultures of the same organisms in the tissue or synovial fluid.
2. Patients who undergo one stage revision surgery for aseptic reasons.

16.4.2 Exclusion Criteria

3. For patients aged <18 years old, synovial fluid is not available through preoperative aspiration or intraoperatively. Patients undergoing a failed one-stage surgery caused by subsequent infection.
4. Patients who have a follow-up period of <1 year. Patients visiting the hospital with antibiotic treatment and cement spacer in their joints and long preoperative history of antibiotic treatment. Patients who have undergone multiple surgeries on the same joint, rheumatoid arthritis and ankylosing spondylitis, serious systemic infection, severe cardiovascular disease, pulmonary system or any other systems, diabetic patients with poor glucose control and malignancies.

The most common definition currently used is one of those proposed by CIAP 2013 criteria, joint fistula are two positive cultures with phenotypically identical MOs, a major criterion that is sufficient to define a diagnosed PJI.

The other minor criteria are following and should have at least three of these minor criteria:

1. Erythrocyte sedimentation rate (ESR) <30 mm for chronic infections and C-reactive protein (CRP level) <10 mg/l for chronic infections or <100 mg/l for acute infections
2. Leukocytes in the synovial fluid (SF) <3000/ul or leukocyte esterase 1+/++
3. Percentage of neutrophils in the synovial fluid (SF) <80%
4. Histology of the periprosthetic tissue with more than five neutrophils in at least five fields at a magnification of 400×
5. Positive culture

These minor criteria are not a gold standard.

16.5 Diagnosis of Periprosthetic Joint Infection

The classical findings are based on clinical symptoms like pain, warm, stiff, and swollen joint. The various other signs are collection, sinus tract, abscess, and necrosis [6–12]. The important drawback is the absence of joint effusions. With these findings, the evaluation of the joint becomes more precise. These FDG PET findings have to be correlated with these various postoperative findings.

16.6 Principle of FDG PET in the Periprosthetic Joint Infection

Leukocytes are activated and show the amount of glucose energy with the expression of glucose transporters [13–15]. The affinity of glucose transporters has to be increased by various cytokines and growth factors. The FDG is transported into the cells by glucose transporters and is phosphorylated to 18F FDG 6 phosphate.

Diagnostic performance of FDG PET-CT in the evaluation of hip and knee replacements. A meta-analysis of one of the studies shows the hip prosthesis as 86% (95% CI), 80–90% and pooled sensitivity of 93% for hip prosthesis [9, 16–20] (Figs. 16.1, 16.2, 16.3, 16.4, 16.5 and 16.6).

16.7 Role of FDG PET in Other Prosthetic Joints

Shoulder replacement is not common but increasing day by day [21]. The common cause in the shoulder is hematoma formation. FDG is not that sensitive.

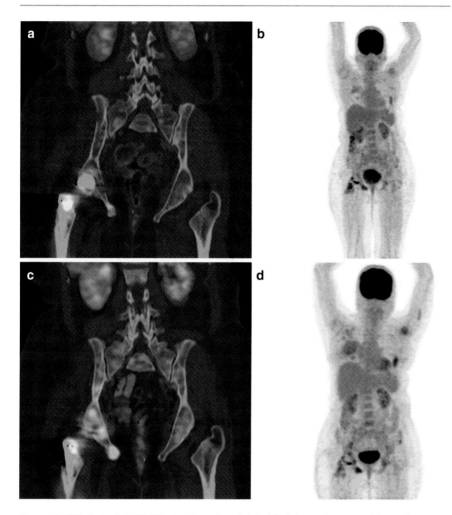

Fig. 16.1 Whole-body PET-CT after 3 weeks of right hip joint replacement. The patient came with a history of pain in the right hip. PET-CT fused images (**a, c**) show a mild focal area of activity in the region of the implant placement in the right femoral shaft. PET images (**b, d**) show uptake in the corresponding region

16.8   Future Perspective

The diagnostic performance of FDG PET in detecting hip and knee joint infection is significantly high [3, 22–27]. With the standardization of acquisition protocols, diagnostic criteria, and reference standard performance of FDG PET can be seen in the future. One of the limitations is the anatomic detail and soft-tissue contrast which cannot be as sensitive on CT compared to MR. The upcoming PET-MR will be an added asset for the evaluation of PJI as it will be having remarkably high sensitivity due to soft tissue contrast.

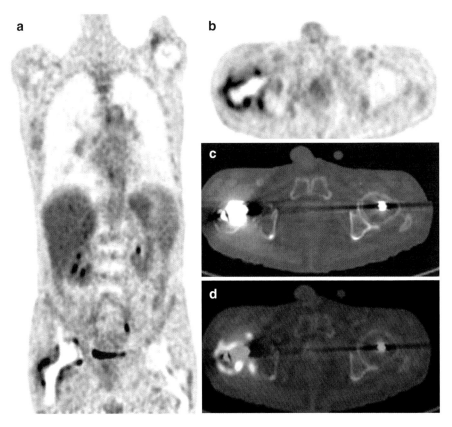

Fig. 16.2 Whole-body PET-CT after 2 months showing the irregular uptake seen in the implant site along the right femoral neck. The patient presented with pain in the right hip region. CT image (**c**) showing metallic artifacts, PET images (**a**, **b**) and fused PET-CT image (**d**) showing diffuse increased linear uptake along the neck consistent with the infection along the prosthesis

16.9 Discussion

Early detection is important. The newer definition of prosthetic joint infections and its modified version is based on a scoring system due to various indicators. The other aspect is to differentiate between the septic and aseptic causes and of the chronic and low-grade infections, but with PET-CT this can be evaluated with better results.

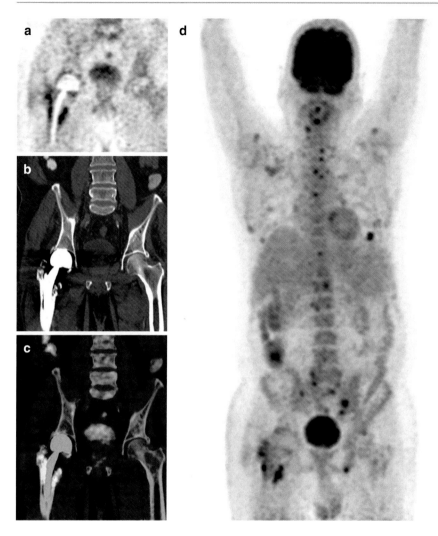

Fig. 16.3 Whole-body PET-CT post right prosthesis 6 weeks with a history of right hip pain and fever on and off. CT shows image (**b**) shows no significant changes. Fused image (**c**) shows linear uptake along the post-prosthesis placement in the femoral shaft. PET images (**a**) and (**d**) showing linear uptake with SUV max of 4.8 consistent with infection

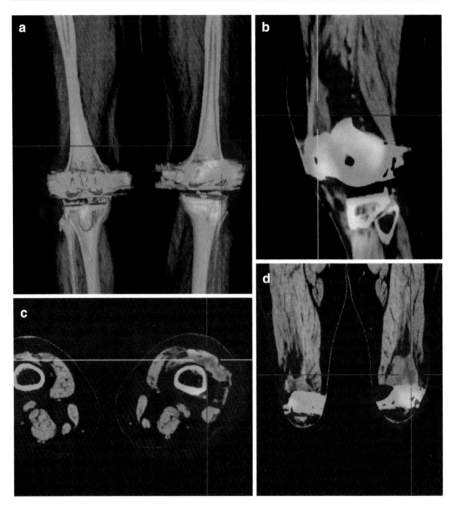

Fig. 16.4 Limited knee joint PET-CT post-prosthesis on both sides. Reformatted image (**a**) and Fused images (**b**), (**c**) and (**d**) showing irregular collection in the suprapatellar location suggestive of infective focus

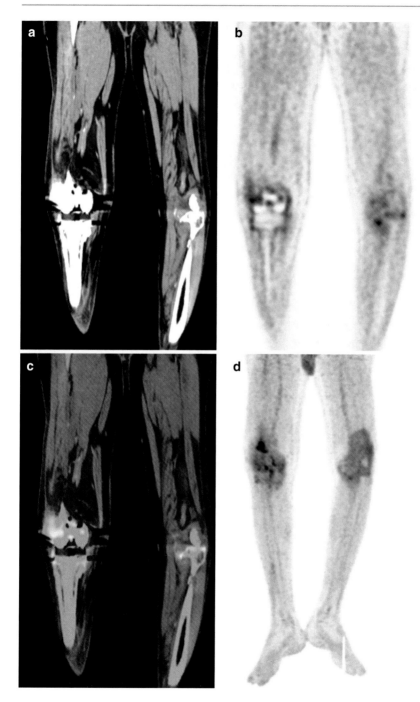

Fig. 16.5 Limited PET-CT both knee joints. Knee replacement right knee. CT image (**a**) showing artifacts. PET images (**b**) and (**d**) show mild area of uptake surrounding the knee joint. Fused PET-CT image (**c**) showing mild uptake consistent with inflammatory changes

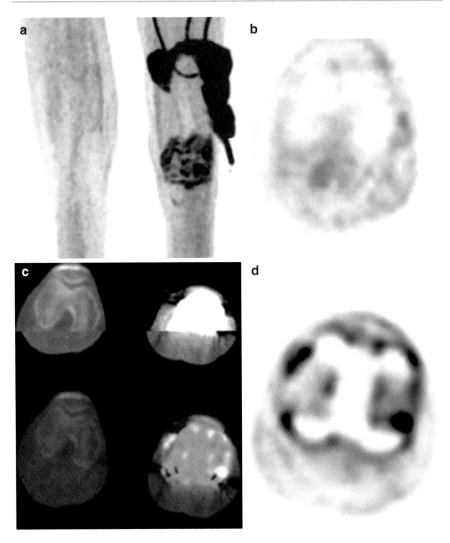

Fig. 16.6 Left knee joint replacement showing irregular areas of uptake surrounding the knee joint with SUV max of 5.2. CT image (**c**) and fused PET-CT image (**a**, **b**, **d**) showing metallic artifacts

16.10 Summary

The diagnosis of prosthetic joint infection is important and challenging. With the availability of PET-CT, the role of the joint prosthesis evaluation is significantly increasing.

Disclosure authors have nothing to disclose.

References

1. Parvizi J, Gehrke T, Mont MA, et al. Introduction: proceedings of international consensus on orthopedic infections. J Arthroplasty. 2019;34:S1–2.
2. Saeed K, McLaren AC, Schwarz EM, et al. The 2018 international consensus meeting on musculoskeletal infection: summary from the Biofilm Workgroup and consensus on biofilm related musculoskeletal infections. J Orthop Res. 2019;37:1007. https://doi.org/10.1002/jor.24229.
3. Amanatullah D, Dennis D, Oltra EG, et al. Hip and knee section, diagnosis, definitions: proceedings of international consensus on orthopedic infections. J Arthroplasty. 2019;34:S329–37.
4. Parvizi J, Tan TL, Goswami K, et al. The 2018 definition of periprosthetic hip and knee infection: an evidence-based and validated criteria. J Arthroplast. 2018;33:1309–14.
5. Toms AD, Davidson D, Masri BA, Duncan CP. The management of peri-prosthetic infection in total joint arthroplasty. J Bone Joint Surg Br. 2006;88:149–55.
6. Parvizi J, Ghanem E, Menashe S, Barrack RL, Bauer TW. Periprosthetic infection: what are the diagnostic challenges? J Bone Joint Surg Am. 2006;88(Suppl 4):138–47.
7. Stumpe KD, Romero J, Ziegler O, Kamel EM, von Schulthess GK, et al. The value of FDG-PET in patients with painful total knee arthroplasty. Eur J Nucl Med Mol Imaging. 2006;33:1218–25.
8. Zhuang H, Duarte PS, Pourdehnad M, et al. The promising role of ^{18}F-FDG PET in detecting infected lower limb prosthesis implants. J Nucl Med. 2001;42:44–8.
9. Manthey N, Reinhard P, Moog F, et al. The use of [^{18}F] fluorodeoxyglucose positron emission tomography to differentiate between synovitis, loosening and infection of hip and knee prostheses. Nucl Med Commun. 2002;23:645–53.
10. Stumpe KD, Nötzli HP, Zanetti M, et al. FDG PET for differentiation of infection and aseptic loosening in total hip replacements: comparison with conventional radiography and three-phase bone scintigraphy. Radiology. 2004;231:333–41.
11. García-Barrecheguren E, Rodríguez Fraile M, Toledo Santana G, et al. FDG-PET: a new diagnostic approach in hip prosthetic replacement. Rev Esp Med Nucl. 2007;26:208–20.
12. Zhuang H, Chacko TK, Hickeson M, et al. Persistent non-specific FDG uptake on PET imaging following hip arthroplasty. Eur J Nucl Med Mol Imaging. 2002;29:1328–33.
13. Dumarey N, Egrise D, Blocklet D, Stallenberg B, Remmelink M, Marmol V, Simaeys GV, Jacobs F, Goldman S. Imaging infection with 18 F-FDG-labeled leukocyte PET/CT: initial experience in 21 patients. J Nucl Med. 2006;47:625–32.
14. Pellegrino D, Bonab AA, Dragotakes SC, Pitman JT, Mariani G, Carter EA. Inflammation and infection: imaging properties of ^{18}F-FDG-labeled white blood cells versus ^{18}F-FDG. J Nucl Med. 2005;46:1522–30.
15. Glaudemans AW, Vries EF, de Galli F, Dierckx RA, Slart RH, Signore A. The use of 18F-FDG-PET/CT for diagnosis and treatment monitoring of inflammatory and infectious diseases. Clin Dev Immunol. 2013;2013:623036.
16. MaraditKremers H, Larson DR, Crowson CS, et al. Prevalence of total hip and knee replacement in the United States. J Bone Joint Surg Am. 2015;97:1386–97.
17. Kapadia BH, Berg RA, Daley JA, et al. Periprosthetic joint infection. Lancet. 2016;387:386–94.

18. Alp E, Cevahir F, Ersoy S, et al. Incidence and economic burden of prosthetic joint infections in a university hospital: a report from a middle-income country. J Infect Public Health. 2016;9:494–8.
19. Charette RS, Melnic CM. Two-stage revision arthroplasty for the treatment of prosthetic joint infection. Curr Rev Musculoskelet Med. 2018;11:332–40.
20. Tande AJ, Patel R. Prosthetic joint infection. Clin Microbiol Rev. 2014;27:302–45.
21. Kwee RM, Broos WA, Brans B, et al. Added value of 18F-FDG PET/CT in diagnosing infected hip pros-thesis. Acta Radiol. 2018;59:569–76.
22. Parvizi J, Tan TL, Goswami K, et al. The 2018 definition of periprosthetic hip and knee infection: an evidence-based and validated criteria. J Arthroplasty. 2018;33:1309–14.
23. Ali F, Wilkinson JM, Cooper JR, et al. Accuracy of joint aspiration for the preoperative diagnosis of infection in total hip arthroplasty. J Arthroplasty. 2006;21:221–6.
24. Signore A, Sconfienza LM, Borens O, et al. Consensus document for the diagnosis of prosthetic joint infections: a joint paper by the EANM, EBJIS, and ESR (with ESCMID endorsement). Eur J Nucl Med Mol Imaging. 2019;46:971–88.
25. Vanquickenborne B, Maes A, Nuyts J, et al. The value of (18)FDG-PET for the detection of infected hip prosthesis. Eur J Nucl Med Mol Imaging. 2003;30(5):705–15.
26. Aydin A, Yu JQ, Zhuang H, et al. Patterns of 18F-FDG PET images in patients with uncomplicated total hip arthroplasty. Hell J Nucl Med. 2015;18:93–6.
27. Verberne SJ, Temmerman OPP, Vuong BH, et al. Fluorodeoxyglucose positron emission tomography imaging for diagnosing periprosthetic hip infection: the importance of diagnostic criteria. Int Orthop. 2018;42:2025–34.

PET-CT in Urological Infections and Inflammations

17

Key Points

Urological infections and inflammations are one of the important causes of pyrexia of unknown origin. The various infections are renal, urinary bladder, Prostate, and rarely ureter and urethra. The major important cause is the renal cause of infections. Renal infections are the most common cause of pyrexia of unknown origin. With the advent of technological advancements, lots of studies are being done to evaluate the renal pathologies especially infection and inflammation and in the settings of pyrexia of unknown origin and patient with underlying renal disease. The diagnosis of acute parenchymal changes like tubulointerstitial nephritis, retroperitoneal fibrosis, acute pyelonephritis, acute glomerulonephritis, acute infections in the settings of pyrexia of unknown origin, and renal cysts with associated infection. Other important causes are Prostatitis, Cystitis, urethral and ureteric infections. PET-CT plays an important role in the evaluation of this infection and inflammation.

17.1   Introduction

Genitourinary infections are one of the common causes of fever [1]. In the settings of pyrexia of unknown origin, renal disease is one of the most common cause for a large number of morbidities and mortalities. With the available imaging modalities like conventional radiography, ultrasound, CT scan, and MRI which are used for the evaluation of various conditions and pathologies associated with urinary obstruction, renal artery stenosis, renal vein thrombosis, and renal infarction [2] (Kidney disease—1). The other important aspects of renal pathology are cystic renal diseases, renal masses causing various pathogenesis which can be infective inflammatory, benign, and malignant conditions. A lot of noninvasive imaging modalities like gallium scanning was done to evaluate the acute tubulointerstitial nephritis which are more prone to renal complications and may ultimately land up into renal failure, i.e., chronic kidney disease. The other imaging modalities like CT and MRI are

© The Author(s), under exclusive license to Springer Nature
Singapore Pte Ltd. 2021
S. Shaikh, *PET-CT in Infection and Inflammation*,
https://doi.org/10.1007/978-981-15-9801-2_17

having problems related to IV contrast which may cause acute kidney disease [3]. Ultrasound is not much specific to evaluate renal pathologies. However, with advancements of ultrasound technology, ultrasound contrast agents, and additional advantage of color Doppler and with all these advancements, the functional status of the kidney cannot be evaluated completely.

17.2   PET-CT Techniques

FDG PET-CT scan is the promising imaging modality to evaluate varieties of Urogenital pathologies like malignancy, metastases, infectious inflammatory conditions, and benign pathologies. Along with the diagnosis, monitoring response to therapy can also be evaluated by PET-CT with incredibly good sensitivity and specificity [4, 5]. The main focus is on the conditions as described above. Usually, PET-CT is done after injecting the FDG as a radiotracer. The CT part is usually done after injecting nonionic IV contrast. For this, the basic criterion is to evaluate the renal parameters which should be in the normal range if elevated, then this IV contrast cannot be done. As a protocol in our Yashoda Hospitals, Hyderabad, we give IV contrast to all the patients except with elevated renal parameters, pediatric age group, and noncooperative patients.

In some of the cases, triphasic intravenous contrast will be given to evaluate the excretion part of the pelviureteric junction in the settings of the obstructions. The advantage of CT is to evaluate the focus of enhancement or non-enhancing areas, pattern of enhancement in various phases. Usually, CT with IV contrast is done in venous phases [6]. However, for any suspected pathologies where characterization is important, triphasic IV contrast study is advisable, i.e., arterial phase, venous phase, and delayed phase. PET-CT plays an important role in the evaluation of difficult conditions.

17.3   PET-CT in Renal Pathologies

17.3.1 PET-CT in Acute Tubulointerstitial Nephritis

The kidney shows a mild increase in size and increased echogenicity (in ultrasound) with a subtle increase or no changes in the echogenicity of the kidney. The role of PET-CT is to evaluate the amount of renal injury based on increased FDG uptake secondary to the presence of lymphocytes, macrophages, neutrophage, and fibro blasts of inflammatory lesions [7–9].

17.3.2 PET-CT in Retroperitoneal Fibrosis

Retroperitoneal fibrosis consists of a group of rare diseases that are characterized by the proliferation of inflammatory tissue most commonly in the infrarenal segment of the abdominal aorta, IVC and along the iliac vessels [10]. This retroperitoneal fibrosis may involve the adjacent ureter causing proximal urinary obstruction and obstructive uropathy symptoms. The other common causes of retroperitoneal fibrosis are lymphoma, retroperitoneal sarcoma, carcinoid tumors, tuberculosis, histoplasmosis, actinomycosis, major abdominal surgeries, retroperitoneal hematoma/hemorrhage, and radiation therapy. Clinically retroperitoneal fibrosis is a nonspecific clinical symptom, and clinical examination is also nonspecific most of the times [11, 12]. With these nonspecific signs and symptoms and nonspecific laboratory tests, the retroperitoneal fibrosis may cause significant renal injuries. The commonest complication is CKD. PET-CT provides important information in the diagnosis, metabolic activity of the lesions in the retroperitoneum. PET also has the advantage to evolve the inflammatory changes along the vascular and perivascular regions. With this advantage of PET scan is assessing the metabolic activity of retroperitoneal tissue [13–15].

17.3.3 PET-CT in Polycystic Kidney Disease

The incidence of cyst involving liver and kidney with infection in polycystic kidney disease is <15% [16, 17]. The various challenges in this entity are nonspecific symptoms, normal kidney and liver function test, and culture tests appearing normal. PET-CT plays an important role in the evaluation of this polycystic kidney disease and can diagnose cyst infections, pyocysts to differentiate between cystic and non-cystic causes of abdominal pain, to differentiate between cyst infection and cyst hemorrhage, to monitoring response to therapy [18, 19]. One of the important advantages of FDG is that it has no nephrotoxicity and hepatotoxicity. Thus, PET-CT is a powerful and same diagnostic tool when used in combination with clinical and biochemical criteria to identify the infection in the cysts (Fig. 17.1).

17.3.4 CKD (Chronic Kidney Disease)

Recently, PET plays an important role in differentiating malignant and benign lesions. This is more relevant to differentiate between cystic lesions with solid components and to differentiate between infected cyst versus cystic renal cell carcinoma. As discussed, PET-CT is more size-dependent and needs to differentiate between infection versus malignancy. The monitoring response to treatment where there is complete/partial resolution of infective inflammatory foci [20, 21] (Fig. 17.2).

17.3.5 PET-CT in Pyelonephritis

Pyelonephritis has two entities: acute pyelonephritis and chronic pyelonephritis. Acute pyelonephritis is the same entity where there is a mild increase in the size of the kidney with an associated mild increase in uptake compared to baseline uptake. Here, it has to be more specific as already radiological uptake will

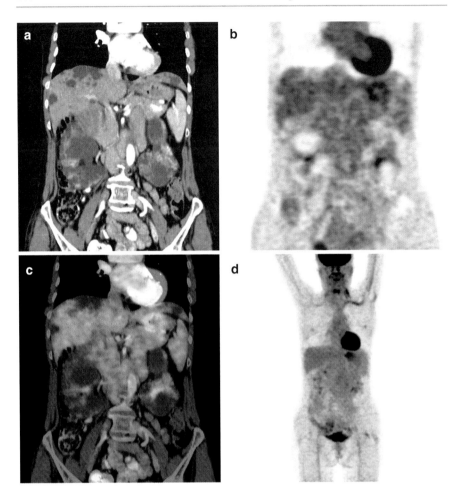

Fig. 17.1 Whole-body PET-CT for evaluation of nonspecific complaints showing CT image (**a**) showing multiple cysts in both lobes of liver and both kidneys, suggestive of polycystic kidney disease. PET image (**b**) and (**d**) showing no uptake in the cysts. Fused image (**c**) also showing no uptake

be there. If possible, dual point imaging is an important entity to differentiate or to categorize a better way. The amount of FDG uptake is directly proportional to the amount of active inflammation [22, 23]. In chronic pyelonephritis, the size of the kidney is small in size and is directly proportional to the chronicity of pyelonephritis. Again, the amount of uptake signifies the infective focus in the renal parenchyma. One of the important differentials is to differentiate between renal infarct and pyelonephritis. The delayed dual point imaging is very helpful in differentiation of the doubtful cases. The amount of SUV uptake is proportional to the FDG uptake [24] (Fig. 17.3).

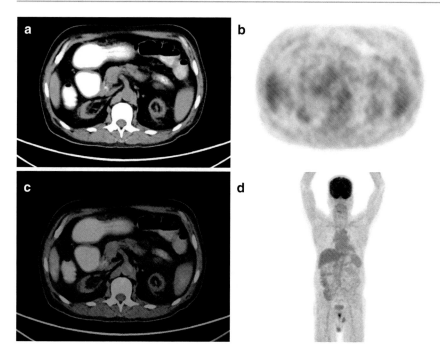

Fig. 17.2 Whole-body PET-CT at the level of showing contracted small-sized kidneys seen on CT image (**a**) with no abnormal metabolic activity seen on PET images (**b, d**) and fused image (**c**) suggestive of renal parenchymal disease

17.3.6 PET-CT in Infected Cyst

The PET-CT plays an important role in evaluating the infective focus in the cyst to differentiate between the cystic RCC versus infected focus in the cyst [25]. Sometimes, the hemorrhagic cyst or hemorrhagic component can be infected which shows diffuse increased uptake [26]. This has to be differentiated from the other differentials by the advent of FDG uptake and dual point imaging (Figs. 17.4 and 17.5).

17.3.7 PET-CT in Renal Injuries

Renal injuries as such do not show any uptake unless and until reactive changes are there [27]. The most important education in renal injury is based on the type of injury. Renal contusion shows an area of focal defect in uptake. Renal laceration does not show any significant pattern of uptake. However, any type of renal injury with associated infection shows increased FDG uptake [28, 29]. The different presentations are perinephric fat stranding, perinephric collections, perinephric abscess, or any combination of this.

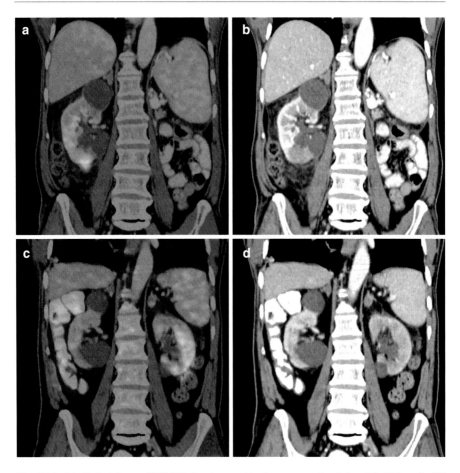

Fig. 17.3 Limited abdomen PET-CT showing cyst in the upper pole of the right kidney in CT image (**b, d**) with no metabolic activity on fused images (**a, c**). The lower pole of the right kidney shows a focal area of hypodense non-enhancing lesion on CT image (**b**) with mild FDG uptake on fused image (**a**) with SUV max of 3.8 suggestive of focal pyelonephritis

17.3.8 Renal Tuberculosis

Renal tuberculosis is one of the important causes of tuberculosis in the Indian sub-continent [30]. Varying stages of tuberculosis involvement is seen. The amount of FDG uptake depends on the acute, subacute, and chronic phases of tuberculosis. Again, the involvement of the perinephric region, pelviureteric junction, and upper ureter can be diagnosed easily. The renal tuberculosis manifests clinically with many other pathological entities like lymphoma, pyelonephritis, fungal infections, collagen diseases, and sometimes metabolic diseases. The role of FDG is to evaluate the amount of uptake, to characterize the lesion, and most important to evaluate the response to treatment. Along with these disease findings, the associated complications also can be evaluated by the PET-CT [31, 32].

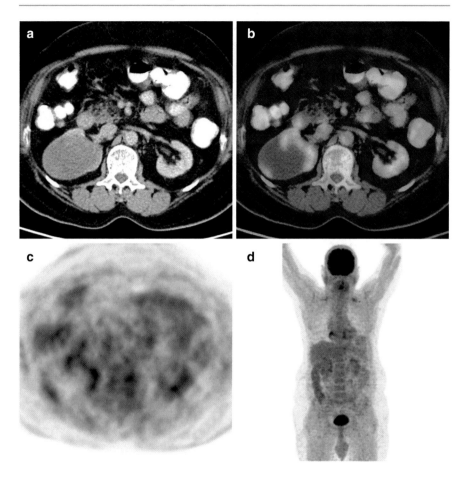

Fig. 17.4 Whole-body PET-CT at the level of kidneys showing cyst in the right kidney with subtle hyperdensity on CT image (**a**). No metabolic activity noted on fused image (**b**) and PET images (**c**, **d**) suggestive of complex cyst

17.4   PET-CT in Ureteric Pathologies

Ureter

Ureteric infections are not as common as renal infections [33]. Ureter is involved in the coexisting renal infections. Primary renal infections are rare except for the tuberculosis or superadded by the obstructive changes in the ureter [34]. PET-CT has an important role in these settings which show subtle ureteric wall enhancement in the intravenous contrast study on CT which corresponds with the increased FDG uptake in these areas. The amount of the uptake is also directly proportional to the amount of the infective load. This sometimes needs to be differentiated from transitional cell carcinoma [35, 36].

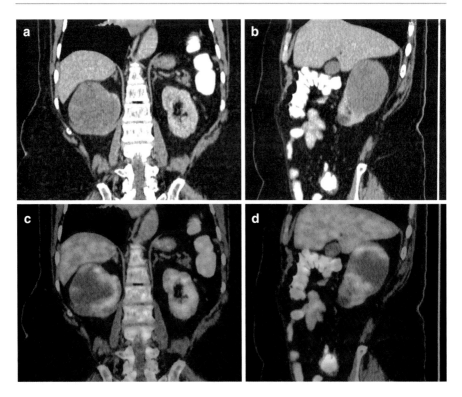

Fig. 17.5 Whole-body PET-CT at the level of kidneys showing cyst in the right kidney with subtle hyperdensity CT images (**a**, **b**). No metabolic activity noted on fused images (**c**, **d**) suggestive of complex cyst

17.5   PET-CT in Urinary Bladder

The urinary bladder is the second most important cause of urinary tract infection [37]. This is represented with direct infection in the urinary bladder or secondary to neurogenic bladder [38]. The important point here is the role of FDG to differentiate between the focal urinary bladder wall thickening and focal transitional cell carcinoma. This plays a very crucial role in the differentiation. In some cases where it is difficult to differentiate then the dual point imaging will be helpful to differentiate based on the SUV Max values. The neurogenic bladder is also an important cause to evaluate the superadded urinary bladder. The other pathologies are tuberculosis, schistosomiasis, Gram-negative organisms, and other causes where PET-CT has an important role for the evaluation [39–41].

The ideal protocol for the evaluation of urinary bladder will be in the delayed phase after a whole-body PET-CT scan when the urinary bladder is well distended. If not, then Lasix can be given for evaluation [42]. The well distended urinary bladder is important

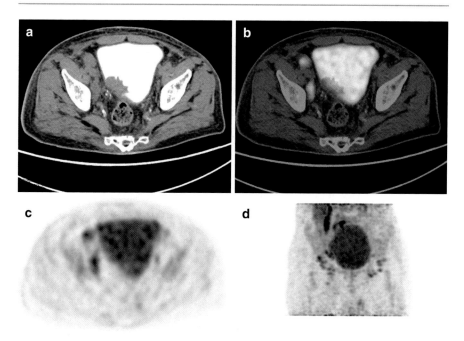

Fig. 17.6 Delayed limited PET-CT of pelvis showing irregular nodular lesion on CT image (**a**). No metabolic activity in PET images (**c, d**) and PET-CT image (**b**) shows no uptake. Mild metabolic activity adjacent right external iliac node with SUV max of 3.5. Findings suggestive of infective etiology. Histopathology confirmed tuberculosis

especially in the cases of subtle focal urinary bladder wall thickening and in situ carcinoma. Peri vesical fat stranding is also an important component to evaluate as this is involved in the infections and in urinary bladder malignancies (Figs. 17.6 and 17.7).

17.6 Prostate

Prostatic infections are more common in the younger age groups [43].The prostate size and attenuation will be normal. PET-CT plays an important role in the evaluation of diffuse prostatitis, prostatic abscess, and other inflammatory pathologies. The important role of PET-CT will be to differentiate between focal prostatitis and prostatic malignancies [43, 44]. Here one important finding is that FDG is avid for prostatic malignancies. For this, PSMA is the important newer radiotracer for the evaluation of prostatic malignancies [45]. In cases of the doubtful SUV Max, the delayed dual point imaging is done for differentiation between both of them. Tuberculosis involving the prostate is also equally common in our Indian subcontinent [46] (Figs. 17.8, 17.9 and 17.10).

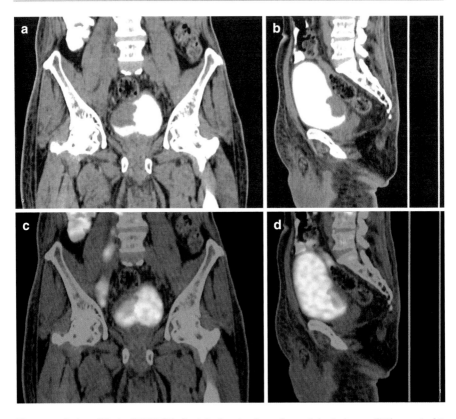

Fig. 17.7 Delayed limited PET-CT of pelvis showing irregular nodular lesion on CT image (**a, b**). No metabolic activity in PET-CT fused images (**c, d**) shows no uptake. Mild metabolic activity adjacent right external iliac node with SUV max of 3.5. Findings suggestive of infective etiology. Histopathology confirmed tuberculosis

Fig. 17.8 Whole-body PET-CT at the level of prostate was showing no CT abnormality. Subtle nodular uptake on PET and fused image (**A**) on the right lateral lobe of the prostate

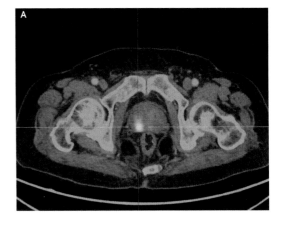

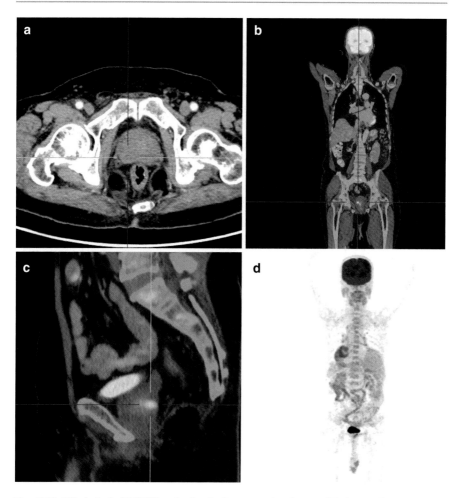

Fig. 17.9 Whole-body PET-CT at the level of prostate showing no CT abnormality image (**a**). Subtle nodular uptake on PET-CT fused images (**b, c**) on the right lateral lobe of the prostate

17.7   Urethra

Urethral infections are not as common; still, PET-CT has important findings [46]. The urethral involvement in tuberculosis is also important [47, 48]. The urethral tumors and infections need to be differentiated from the focal urethral infections.

17.8   Penis

Penile infections are less common as compared to the other urogenital infections [49]. Most of these infections are related to the sexually transmitted diseases, especially the human papillomavirus. FDG PET-CT definitely has an important role in

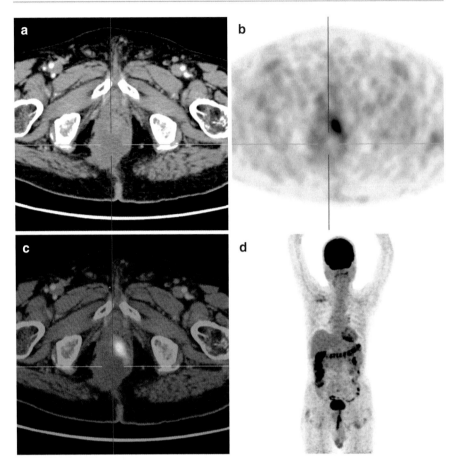

Fig. 17.10 Whole-body PET-CT, CT image showing irregular hypodensity in the periprostatic on right side seen in CT image (**a**) suggestive of periprostatic abscess. PET (**b, d**) and fused images (**c**) showing focal nodular uptake on the left side suggestive of viable infective tissue

the evaluation of these infections; however, the penile cancers need to be distinguished [50].

17.9 Epididymo-Orchitis

Epididymo-orchitis is the commonest infection and inflammation of the male genital tract. PET-CT plays an important role in the evaluation by showing diffuse uptake. The common causes are tuberculosis and infective foci. Sometimes Epididymo-orchitis very difficult to differentiate from the foal testicular neoplasms [51, 52].

17.10 Infections of Female Genital Tract

The infections of the female genital tract are common. The commonest presentation of this is in the form of pelvic inflammatory disease, salpingo-oophoritis, and endometrial tuberculosis. FDG PET-CT plays an important role in the evaluation showing increased uptake. Endometrial tuberculosis needs to be differentiated from endometrial carcinoma [53, 54].

17.11 Conclusion

Pyrexia of unknown origin is one of the important broad entities, whereby doing a whole-body PET-CT it is easily possible to diagnose the lesion, characterize the lesion, associated complications, and monitoring response to treatment. This also applies specifically to the urogenital system. FDG PET-CT is most widely used for the evaluation of the urogenital infections and inflammation. PSMA is only used for the evaluation of prostatic carcinomas.

References

1. Foxman B, Barlow R, D'arcy H, Gillespie B, Sobel JD. Urinary tract infection: self-reported incidence and associated costs. Ann Epidemiol. 2000;10(8):509–15.
2. Sorensen SM, Schonheyder HC, Nielsen H. The role of imaging of the urinary tract in patients with urosepsis. Int J Infect Dis. 2013;17:e299–303.
3. McCullough PA. Contrast-induced acute kidney injury. J Am Coll Cardiol. 2008;51:1419–28.
4. Basu S, Chryssikos T, Moghadam-Kia S, Zhuang H, Torigian DA, Alavi A. Positron emission tomography as a diagnostic tool in infection: present role and future possibilities. Semin Nucl Med. 2009;39(1):36–51.
5. Balink H, Collins J, Bruyn G, Gemmel F. F-18 FDG PET/CT in the diagnosis of fever of unknown origin. Clin Nucl Med. 2009;34(12):862–8.
6. Kekelidze M, Dwarkasing RS, Dijkshoorn ML, et al. Kidney and urinary tract imaging: triple-bolus multidetector CT urography as a one-stop shop—protocol design, opacification, and image quality analysis. Radiology. 2010;255:508–16.
7. McCammack KC, Hawkes NC, Silverman ED, et al. PET/CT appearance of acute pyelonephritis. Clin Nucl Med. 2013;38:299–301.
8. Katagiri D, Masumoto S, Katsuma A, et al. Positron emission tomography combined with computed tomography (PET-CT) as a new diagnostic tool for acute tubulointerstitial nephritis (AIN) in oliguric or haemodialysedpatients. NDT Plus. 2010;3:155–9.
9. Katagiri D, Masumoto S, Katsuma A, Minami E, Hoshino T, Inoue T, et al. Positron emission tomography combined with computed tomography (PET-CT) as a new diagnostic tool for acute tubulointerstitial nephritis (AIN) in oliguric or haemodialysed patients. NDT Plus. 2010;3(2):155–9.
10. van Bommel EF, Jansen I, Hendriksz TR, Aarnoudse ALHJ. Idiopathic retroperitoneal fibrosis. Medicine (Baltimore). 2009;88:193–201.
11. Scheel PJ, Feeley N. Retroperitoneal fibrosis: the clinical, laboratory, and radiographic presentation. Medicine. 2009;88:202–7.
12. Van Bommel E, Jansen I, Hendriksz T, Aarnoudse A. Idiopathic retroperitoneal fibrosis: prospective evaluation of incidence and clinicoradiologic presentation. Medicine. 2009;88:193–201.

13. Moroni G, Castellani M, Balzani A, et al. The value of (18)F-FDG PET/CT in the assessment of active idiopathic retroperitoneal fibrosis. Eur J Nucl Med Mol Imaging. 2012;39:1635–42.
14. Nakajo M, Jinnouchi S, Tanabe H, Tateno R, Nakajo M. 18F-fluorodeoxyglucose positron emission tomography features of idiopathic retroperitoneal fibrosis. J Comput Assist Tomography. 2007;31:539–43.
15. Jansen I, Hendriksz TR, Han SH, Huiskes AW, van Bommel EF. (18)F-fluorodeoxyglucose position emission tomography (FDG-PET) for monitoring disease activity and treatment response in idiopathic retroperitoneal fibrosis. Eur J Intern Med. 2010;21:216–21.
16. Migali G, Annet L, Lonneux M, Devuyst O. Renal cyst infection in autosomal dominant polycystic kidney disease. Nephrol Dial Transplant. 2008;23:404–5.
17. Bobot M, Ghez C, Gondouin B, et al. Diagnostic performance of (18)F fluorodeoxyglucose positron emission tomography-computed tomography in cyst infection in patients with autosomal dominant polycystic kidney disease. Clin Microbiol Infect. 2016;22:71–7.
18. Paschali AN, Georgakopoulos AT, Pianou NK, et al. 18F-fluorodeoxyglucose positron emission tomography/computed tomography in infected polycystic kidney disease. World J Nucl Med. 2015;14:57–9.
19. Jouret F, Lhommel R, Beguin C, et al. Positron-emission computed tomography in cyst infection diagnosis in patients with autosomal dominant polycystic kidney disease. Clin J Am Soc Nephrol. 2011;6:1644–50.
20. Couser WG, Remuzzi G, Mendis S. The contribution of chronic kidney disease to the global burden of major non-communicable diseases. Kidney Int. 2011;80:1258–70.
21. Ruggenenti P, Cravedi P, Remuzzi G. Mechanisms and treatment of CKD. J Am Soc Nephrol. 2012;23:1917–28.
22. Morelle M, Jaillard A, Bellevre D, Collet G, Petyt G. 18F-FDG PET/CT in renal infections: evidence of acute pyelonephritis in a horseshoe kidney. Clin Nucl Med. 2017;42(2):112–3.
23. Lane DR, Takhar SS. Diagnosis and management of urinary tract infectionand pyelonephritis. Emerg Med Clin North Am. 2011;29:539–52.
24. Zhuang H, Pourdehnad M, Lambright ES, Yamamoto AJ, Lanuti M, Li P, Mozley PD, Rossman MD, Albelda SM, Alavi A. Dual time point ^{18}F-FDG PET imaging for differentiating malignant from inflammatory processes. J Nucl Med. 2001;42:1412–7.
25. Agrawal K, Bhattacharya A, Singh SK, Manohar K, Kashyap R, Mittal BR. Polycystic kidney disease: renal cyst infection detected on F-18 FDG PET/CT. Clin Nucl Med. 2011;36:1122–3.
26. Israel G, Bosniak M. An update of the Bosniak renal cyst classification system. Urology. 2005;66:484–8.
27. Thomas ME, Blaine C, Dawnay A, et al. The definition of acute kidney injury and its use in practice. Kidney Int. 2015;87:62–73.
28. Alonso RC, Nacenta SB, Martinez PD, Guerrero AS, Fuentes CG. Kidney in danger: CT findings of blunt and penetrating renal trauma. Radiographics. 2009;29:2033–53.
29. Ynch TH, Martínez-Piñeiro L, Plas E, Serafetinides E, Türkeri L, Santucci RA, Hohenfellner M. EAU guidelines on urological trauma. Eur Urol. 2005;47:1–15.
30. Gupta NP. Genitourinary tuberculosis. Indian J Urol. 2008;24:355.
31. Kosterink JGW. Positron emission tomography in the diagnosis and treatment management of tuberculosis. Curr Pharm Des. 2011;17:2875–80.
32. Merchant S, Bharati A, Merchant N. Tuberculosis of the genitourinary system-urinary tract tuberculosis: renal tuberculosis-part II. Indian J Radiol Imaging. 2013;23:64–77.
33. Hooton TM. Uncomplicated urinary tract infection. New Engl J Med. 2012;366:1028–37.
34. Cek M, Lenk S, Naber KG, Bishop MC, Johansen TE, Botto H, et al. EAU guidelines for the management of genitourinary tuberculosis. Eur Urol. 2005;48:353–62.
35. Jamar F, Buscombe J, Chiti A, et al. EANM/SNMMI guideline for 18F-FDG use in inflammation and infection. J Nucl Med. 2013;54(4):647–58. https://doi.org/10.2967/jnumed.112.112524.
36. Vaidyanathan S, Patel CN, Scarsbrook AF, Chowdhury FU. FDG PET/CT in infection and inflammation—current and emerging clinical applications. Clin Radiol. 2015;70(7):787–800.
37. Ejrnæs K. Bacterial characteristics of importance for recurrent urinary tract infections caused by *Escherichia coli*. Dan Med Bull. 2011;58:B4187.

38. Nseyo U, Santiago-Lastra Y. Long-term complications of the neurogenic bladder. Urol Clin North Am. 2017;44:355–66.
39. Karanikas G, Beheshti M. (1)(1)C-acetate PET/CT imaging: physiologic uptake, variants, and pitfalls. PET Clin. 2014;9(3):339–44.
40. Walker SJ, Zambon J, Andersson KE, et al. Bladder capacity is a biomarker for a bladder centric versus systemic manifestation in interstitial cystitis/bladder pain syndrome. J Urol. 2017;198(2):369–75. https://doi.org/10.1016/j.juro.2017.02.022.
41. Salem N, Balkman JD, Wang J, et al. In vivo imaging of schistosomes to assess disease burden using positron emission tomography (PET). PLoSNegl Trop Dis. 2010;4(9):e827.
42. Ceriani L, Suriano S, Ruberto T, Giovanella L. Could different hydration protocols affect the quality of ^{18}F-FDG PET/CT images? J Nucl Med Technol. 2011;39:77–82.
43. Kao PF, Chou YH, Lai CW. Diffuse FDG uptake in acute prostatitis. Clin Nucl Med. 2008;33:308–10.
44. Ho L, Quan V, Henderson R, Seto J. High-grade urothelial carcinoma of the prostate on FDG PET-CT. Clin Nucl Med. 2007;32:746–7.
45. Mease RC, Foss CA, Pomper MG. PET imaging in prostate cancer: focus on prostate-specific membrane antigen. Curr Top Med Chem. 2013;13:951–62.
46. Kulchavenya E, Brizhatyuk E, Khomyakov V. Diagnosis and therapy for prostate tuberculosis. Ther Adv Urol. 2014;6:129–34.
47. Metser U, Even-Sapir E. Increased (18)F-fluorodeoxyglucose uptake in benign, non-physiologic lesions found on whole-body positron emission tomography/computed tomography (PET/CT): accumulated data from four years of experience with PET/CT. Semin Nucl Med. 2007;37:206–22.
48. Stelzmueller I, Huber H, Wunn R, Hodolic M, Mandl M, Schinko H, Lamprecht B, Fellner F, Skanjeti A, Giammarile F, Colletti PM, Gabriel M, Rubello D. 18F-FDG PET/CT in the initial assessment and for follow-up in patients with tuberculosis. Clin Nucl Med. 2015;41(4):187–94.
49. Severson J, Evans TY, Lee P, et al. Human papillomavirus infections: epidemiology, pathogenesis, and therapy. J Cutan Med Surg. 2001;5:43–60.
50. Kidd LC, Chaing S, Chipollini J, et al. Relationship between human papilloma virus and penile cancer implications for prevention and treatment. Transl Androl Urol. 2017;6(5):791–802.
51. Ran P, Liang X, Zhang Y, Sun P, Dong A. FDG PET/CT in a case of bilateral tuberculous epididymo-orchitis. Clin Nucl Med. 2019;44(9):757–60.
52. Chopra S, Dharmaraja A. FDG PET/CT images demonstrating epididymo-orchitis in a patient with HIV, acute kidney injury and known epididymo-orchitis on scrotal ultrasound. Clin Nucl Med. 2015;40(2):e171–2.
53. Lerman H, Metser U, Grisaru D, Fishman A, Lievshitz G, Even-Sapir E. Normal and abnormal 18F-FDG endometrial and ovarian uptake in pre- and postmenopausal patients: assessment by PET/CT. J Nucl Med. 2004;45:266–71.
54. Harkirat S, Anana SS, Indrajit LK, Dash AK. Pictorial essay: PET/CT in tuberculosis. Indian J Radiol Imaging. 2008;18(2):141–7.

PET-CT in Viral Infections

18

Key Points

Viral infections are an important clinical entity with varied clinical symptoms and significant overlap with bacterial symptoms. However, some viral conditions have nonspecific symptoms which can be severe enough to cause septicemia.

Viral infections involve all the age groups with common symptoms like fever, common cold, GI symptoms like vomiting, diarrhea, neurological symptoms like headache, confusion, irritation, loss of consciousness. The specific pathological entity has to be defined and differentiated.

18.1 Introduction

PET-CT in viral infections is having a significant role in evaluating the amount or extent of disease, disease burden, disease involvement, and severity of the disease in the affected organs which is quantified by the SUV max value [1]. However, PET-CT cannot differentiate the exact cause and cannot differentiate in the varied overlap findings in malignant and benign conditions [2]. This has relevance in relation to meningitis/encephalitis which can be viral or bacterial or other causes of meningitis.

18.2 Principle of PET-CT

The basic principle of FDG PET is to demonstrate the increased uptake associated findings of nodal involvement, monitoring disease progression, and monitoring response to treatment [3, 4]. The pathological basis of this is a virus infects the body which activates neutrophils, monocytes, and T cells by releasing local chemokines. Thus, in active inflammation, the activated neutrophils are dependent on anaerobic

© The Author(s), under exclusive license to Springer Nature
Singapore Pte Ltd. 2021
S. Shaikh, *PET-CT in Infection and Inflammation*,
https://doi.org/10.1007/978-981-15-9801-2_18

glycolysis requiring increased glucose which is directly proportional to high FDG uptake. Other cell granulocytes and macrophages also play an important role in facilitating glucose transport in chronic conditions. Thus, FDG uptake is directly proportional to the amount of active inflammation.

18.3   Neurological Infections

Subacute Sclerosing Panencephalitis (SSPE) is one of the important components of the neurodegenerative disease [5]. This has features of cognitive and behavioral changes, atonic and/or myoclonic seizures, periodic paroxysms on electroencephalogram (EEG), and increased measles antibodies in cerebrospinal fluid. SSPE is one of the dreadful forms of disease which is caused by the reactivation of the measles virus in the brain for several years after the episode of the primary measles infection. Although it has been studied for many years, its pathogenesis and treatment have not been elucidated. FDG PET-CT is now evolving as an important imaging modality for SSPE [6]. One of the studies by Yeong Seon et al. proved that cortical glucose metabolism is significantly reduced in patients with SSPE, but some of them are normal [7]. The immune system is involved in this pathogenesis. The pattern of FDG PET-CT shows variable uptake patterns depending on the various locations during viral exposure. CNS's presentations are of meningitis, encephalitis, dural enhancement, gyral enhancement and combination of any of this with or without cerebral edema (Figs. 18.1 and 18.2).

18.4   Head and Neck Viral Infections

18.4.1 Upper Respiratory Tract Infection

Upper respiratory tract infection is one of the most common infections. This includes the varied conditions like rhinitis, sinusitis, ear infections, acute pharyngitis, tonsillitis, epiglottitis, and various infections. Laryngitis is one of the important components of the upper respiratory tract involvement. The amount of FDG uptake is directly proportional to the amount and acuteness of infectivity [8–11].

18.4.2 Acute Pharyngitis

Acute pharyngitis is one of the important viral infections in young children. Various mild changes due to clinical sysmptoms are important for the evalaution.

Acute pharyngitis is caused by viruses in more than 70% of cases in young children. Mild pharyngeal redness and swelling and tonsil enlargement are typical. Streptococcal infection is rare in children under five and more common in older

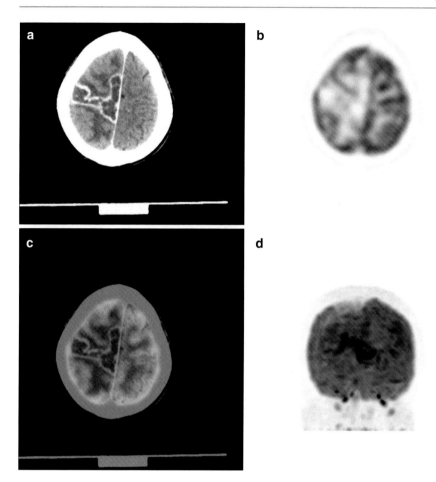

Fig. 18.1 Limited brain PET showing meningeal enhancement on CT image (**a**) in the right high parietal region corresponding PET (**b**) and (**d**) and fused image (**c**) show mild FDG uptake. FDG is not overly sensitive to brain pathology

children. In countries with crowded living conditions and populations that may have a genetic predisposition, post-streptococcal sequelae such as acute rheumatic fever and carditis are common in school-age children but may also occur in those under five. Acute pharyngitis in conjunction with the development of a membrane on the throat is nearly always caused by *Corynebacterium diphtheriae* in developing countries. However, with the almost universal vaccination of infants with the DTP (diphtheria–tetanus–pertussis) vaccine, diphtheria is rare. FDG PET-CT plays an important role in the evaluation of pharyngitis. The amount of uptake is directly proportional to the amount of inflammation [12, 13].

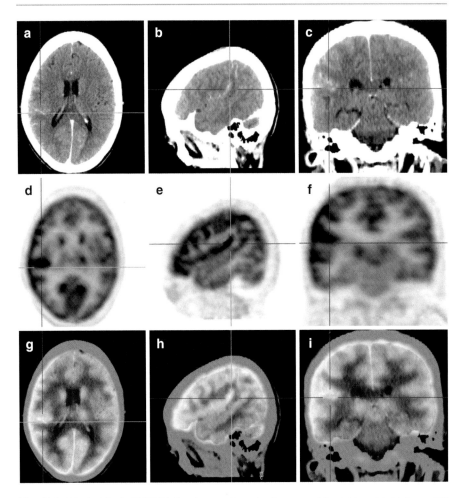

Fig. 18.2 Limited brain PET-CT showing meningeal enhancement in right parietal lobe on CT images (**a**, **b**, **c**) and corresponding PET (**d**, **e**, **f**) and fused images (**g**, **h**, **i**) showing focal area of uptake along the meninges suggestive of meningitis

18.5   Viral Infection in Chest

18.5.1 Viral Infection

Viral infection in the chest has a varied presentation with an overlap of bacteremia. However, the commonest presentation is patchy consolidations. This is again related to upper respiratory tract and lower respiratory tract which are commonly associated with bacterial infections in later stages. SARS and other viral infections commonly present as ARDS (acute respiratory distress syndrome). FDG PET-CT is now

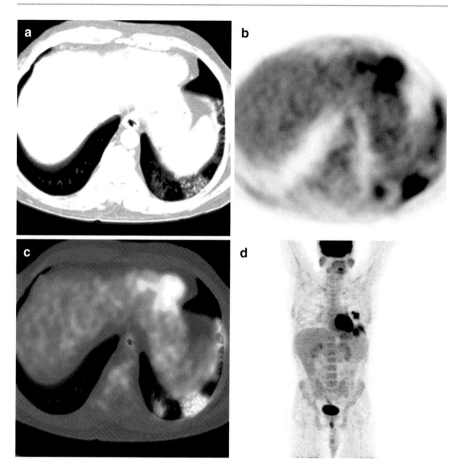

Fig. 18.3 Whole-body PET-CT for high-grade fever showing patchy parenchymal infiltrates in left lower lobe on CT image (**a**). These infiltrates show significant increased uptake with SUV max of 6.5 on PET (**b**) and (**d**) and fused image (**c**) consistent with patchy pneumonitis due to viral infection

an important imaging modality to evaluate various viral infections in the chest [14, 15] (Figs. 18.3, 18.4 and 18.5).

18.5.2 COVID-19

The pathogenesis is similar to other causes. However, bilateral consolidations predominantly peripheral with air bronchogram and pulmonary vessel cut off sign are the hallmark presentations on CT. These findings are clinically consistent with ARDS. A couple of studies on COVID-19 FDG uptake showed the multiorgan involvement with damage especially to GI tract, kidneys, bone marrow, heart, and

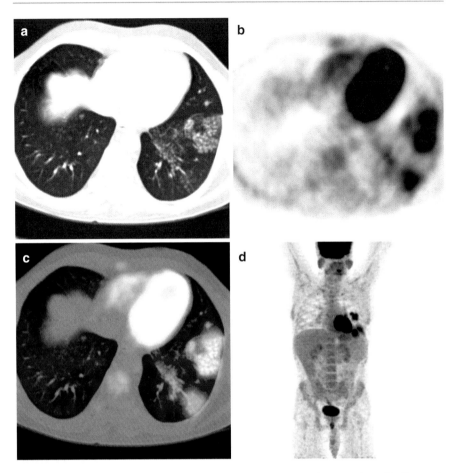

Fig. 18.4 Whole-body PET-CT for high-grade fever showing patchy parenchymal infiltrates in left lower lobe on CT image (**a**). These infiltrates show significant increased uptake with SUV max of 6.5 on PET (**b**) and (**d**) and fused image (**c**) consistent with patchy pneumonitis due to viral infection

other organs. The PET-CT findings are similar to other viral infections. The only advantage is to detect, evaluate the extent, and monitor the response to treatment [16, 17]. Limited imaging is done in this condition. However, the results are correlating with the amount of lung involvement (Figs. 18.6 and 18.7).

18.6   Viral Infections in Abdomen

In early and acute stages, no specific classical findings are there in the GI tract. Liver is one of the commonest organs involved in viral hepatitis especially commonly by Hepatitis-B, Hepatitis-A and C. The FDG presentation depends on the

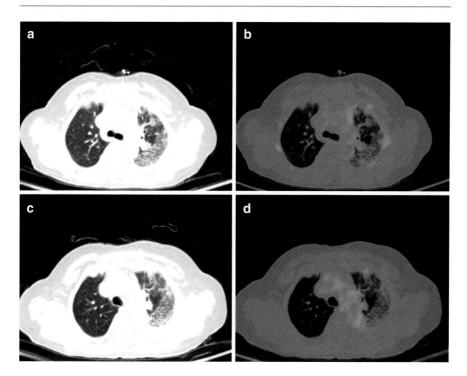

Fig. 18.5 Whole-body PET-CT with images at the level of both the upper lobe of the lung. Inhomogeneous parenchymal opacity with ground glass opacification seen in left upper lobe with focal pleural thickening image (**a**) and (**c**) and minimal FDG uptake in fused images (**b**) and (**d**) suggestive of infective inflammatory pathology

stage of liver involvement (Figs. 18.8 and 18.9). Early stage no change, acute or chronic stage diffuse increased uptake in the liver secondary to Hepatitis, chronic and delayed stages where liver progresses to chronic liver disease or cirrhosis of liver or further may be predisposing to hepatocellular carcinoma. Here FDG PET-CT evaluates the extent of the disease and response to the treatment especially in acute stages which are reversible [12, 18–21]. The other presentations are mild peritoneal thickening. The next common organ involved are the genital organs, cervix in female and penis in male. Ca cervix is due to various predisposing factors and one of them is by various viral infections [22, 23].

The carcinoma penis is one of the predisposing factors caused by HPV (human papilloma virus) [24, 25].

Thus, FDG PET-CT plays an important role in the evaluation of viral infections to detect, extent disease involvement, monitoring disease progression, and treatment outcomes. There are lots of research going on especially in COVID-19 PET-CT evaluation. The findings mentioned in our chapter are based on preliminary research.

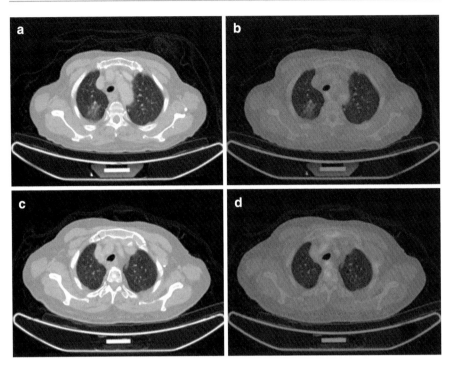

Fig. 18.6 Small patchy pneumonitis apex of right lung in image (**a**, **c**). Fused PET-CT images (**b**) and (**d**) show minimal nonspecific FDG uptake suggestive of infective inflammatory pathology

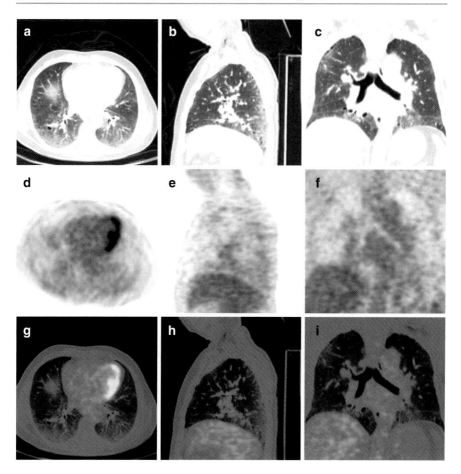

Fig. 18.7 Limited PET-CT chest. CT showing ground-glass opacities right upper lobe and both lower lobes in images (**a**, **b**, and **c**) with minimal uptake on fused (**g**, **h**, **i**) and PET images (**d**, **e**, **f**) suggestive of nonspecific infective pathology

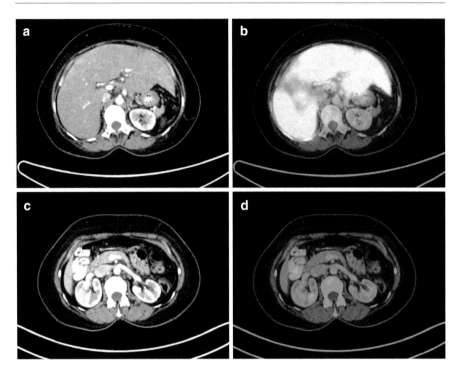

Fig. 18.8 Whole-body PET-CT at the level of abdomen liver showing subtle inhomogenous ena-hancement in liver more in left lobe image (**a**, **c**) diffuse intense uptake involving entire liver parenchyma on PET and PET-CT images (**b**) with SUV max of 13.5. Minimal ill-defined hypoden-sities in both lobes of liver suggestive of hepatitis

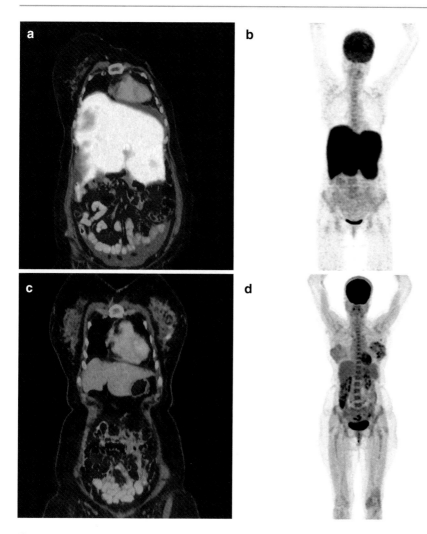

Fig. 18.9 Whole-body PET-CT at the level of abdomen liver showing diffuse intense uptake involving entire liver parenchyma on PET (**b, d**) and PET-CT (**a, c**) images with SUV max of 13.5. Minimal ill-defined hypodensities in both lobes of liver suggestive of hepatitis

References

1. Alauddin MM, Conti PS, Mazza SM, Hamzeh FM, Lever JR. 9-[(3-[^{18}F]-fluoro-1-hydroxy-2-propoxy) methyl] guanine ([^{18}F]-FHPG): a potential imaging agent of viral infection and gene therapy using PET. Nucl Med Biol. 1996;23:787–92.
2. Seemann MD, Seemann O, Luboldt W, et al. Differentiation of malignant from benign solitary pulmonary lesions using chest radiography, spiral CT and HRCT. Lung Cancer. 2000;29:105–24.

3. Basu S, Hess S, Braad P-EN, et al. The basic principles of FDG-PET/CT imaging. PET Clin. 2014;9(4):355–70.
4. Hess S, Blomberg BA, Zhu HJ et al. The Pivotal Role of FDG-PET/CT in Modern Medicine, Academic Radiology, 2014;21(2):232–49.
5. Chaudhuri A, Kennedy PG. Diagnosis and treatment of viral encephalitis. Postgrad Med J. 2002;78:575–83.
6. Yilmaz K, Yilmaz M, Mete A, Celen Z, et al. A correlative study of FDG PET, MRI/CT, electroencephalography, and clinical features in subacute sclerosing panencephalitis. Clin Nucl Med. 2010;35:675–81.
7. Seo Y-S, Kim H-S, Jung D-E. 18F-FDG PET and MRS of the early stages of subacute sclerosing panencephalitis in a child with a normal initial MRI. Pediatr Radio. 2010;40(11):1822–5.
8. Gordon BA, Flanagan FL, Dehdashti F. Whole-body positron emission tomography: normal variations, pitfalls, and technical considerations. Am J Roentgenol. 1997;169:1675–80.
9. Bhargava P, Rahman S, Wendt J. Atlas of confounding factors in head and neck PET/CT imaging. Clin Nucl Med. 2011;36:e20–9.
10. Basu S, Chryssikos T, Moghadam-Kia S, Zhuang H, Torigian DA, Alavi A. Positron emission tomography as a diagnostic tool in infection: present role and future possibilities. Semin Nucl Med. 2009;39(1):36–51. https://doi.org/10.1053/j.semnuclmed.2008.08.004.
11. Simons KS, Pickkers P, Bleeker-Rovers CP, Oyen WJ, Hoeven JG. F-18-fluorodeoxyglucose positron emission tomography combined with CT in critically ill patients with suspected infection. Intensive Care Med 2010;36(3):504–511. doi: https://doi.org/10.1007/s00134-009-1697-8.
12. Jamar F, Buscombe J, Chiti A, Christian PE, Delbeke D, Donohoe KJ, Israel O, Martin Comin J, Signore A. EANM/SNMMI guideline for 18F-FDG use in inflammation and infection. J Nucl Med. 2013;54(4):647–58.
13. Vaidyanathan S, Patel CN, Scarsbrook AF, Chowdhury FU. FDG PET/CT in infection and inflammation current and emerging clinical applications. Clin Radiol. 2015;70(7):787–800.
14. Takalkar AM, Bruno GL, Makanjoula AJ, El-Haddad G, Lilien DL, Payne DK. A potential role for F-18 FDG PET/CT in evaluation and management of fibrosing mediastinitis. Clin Nucl Med. 2007;32(9):703–6.
15. Capitanio S, Nordin AJ, Noraini AR, Rossetti C. PET/CT in non-oncological lung diseases: current applications and future perspectives. Eur Respir Rev. 2016;25:247–58.
16. hefer S, Thomasson D, Seidel J, Reba RC, Bohannon JK, Lackemeyer MG, et al. Modeling [(18)F]-FDG lymphoid tissue kinetics to characterize nonhuman primate immune response to Middle East respiratory syndrome-coronavirus aerosol challenge. EJNMMI Res. 2015;5:65.
17. Qin C, Liu F, Yen TC, Lan X. 18F-FDG PET/CT findings of COVID-19: a series of four highly suspected cases. Eur J Nucl Med Mol Imaging. 2020;47:1281.
18. Koff G, Sterbis JR, Davison JM, Montilla-Soler JL. A unique presentation of appendicitis: F-18 FDG PET/CT. Clin Nucl Med. 2006;31(11):704–6.
19. European Association for the Study of the Liver. EASL clinical practice guidelines on the management of ascites, spontaneous bacterial peritonitis, and hepatorenal syndrome in cirrhosis. J Hepatol. 2010;53:397–417.
20. Li XJ, Li FQ, Han JK, et al. Ascites metabolism measurement enhanced the diagnostic value and accuracy of prognostic evaluation in 18F-FDG PET/CT studies in malignant ascites patients. Nucl Med Commun. 2013;34:544–50.
21. Kim MJ, Kim YS, Cho YH, Jang HY, Song JY, Lee SH, et al. Use of 18F-FDG PET to predict tumor progression and survival in patients with intermediate hepatocellular carcinoma treated by trans-arterial chemo-embolization. Korean J Intern Med. 2015;30:308–15.
22. Hariri S, Unger ER, Sternberg M, et al. Prevalence of genital human papillomavirus among females in the United States, the National Health and Nutrition Examination Survey, 2003–2006. J Infect Dis. 2011;204:566–73.

23. Kidd EA, Siegel BA, Dehdashti F, et al. The standardized uptake value for F-18 fluorodeoxy-glucose is a sensitive predictive biomarker for cervical cancer treatment response and survival. Cancer. 2007;110(8):1738–44.
24. Scher B, Seitz M, Reiser M, Hungerhuber E, Hahn K, Tiling R. Herzog 18F-FDG PET/CT for staging of penile cancer. J Nucl Med. 2005;46:1460–5.
25. Ottenhof SR, Vegt E. The role of PET/CT imaging in penile cancer. Trans Androl Urol. 2017;6(5):833–8.

PET-CT in the Organ Transplantation

19

Key Points
Solid-organ transplant is one of the reserved therapeutic options for end-stage diseases involving the solid organs. The follow-up of transplant patients depends on the short-term and long-term presentations. The problem with organ transplantation is that the biological tests and various imaging techniques are nonspecific. Infection and inflammation are the two common complications after solid organ transplantation. These conditions are of not much relevance clinically. Even the routine Conventional Imaging modalities are more important than this. FDG PET-CT is an important modality to evaluate pre-transplant and posttransplant status. PET-CT also helps in the evaluation of infections and probably one of the important causes of rejection.

19.1 Introduction

With the advent of advancements in the medical field, the chances of any end-stage organ failure landing as an end-stage disease is quite common due to early diagnosis of these processes. This is because of a pre-existing infection that is dormant and cannot be picked up by any other imaging modalities. FDG PET also plays an important role in the posttransplant infection scenario [1–3]. This is one of the important aspects of organ transplant to develop complications after transplantation. This is due to immunosuppressive therapy which is administered after transplantation [4].

19.2 PET-CT in Organ Transplantation

Organ transplantation is the last alternative for end-stage organ diseases, especially of solid organs. Organ transplantation is a crucial part of the normal functioning of the organs after the transplantation. The most important and common analysis of

© The Author(s), under exclusive license to Springer Nature
Singapore Pte Ltd. 2021
S. Shaikh, *PET-CT in Infection and Inflammation*,
https://doi.org/10.1007/978-981-15-9801-2_19

post-organ transplant is the complications after transplantation. These complications can be minor to major which needs to be differentiated. The most common and important complication is the opportunistic infections, and in severe cases, it can be transplant rejection. There are many causes for the posttransplant evaluation. Since the routine conventional imaging modalities like X-ray, ultrasound, CT, and MRI are important but the early changes of the infection cannot be evaluated. PET-CT is only the imaging modality which demonstrates the focus of infection and the organ involved. The amount of FDG uptake is the indicator of this. However, in later stages, the organ rejection can also be evaluated. One of the most severe complications of reduced immunity is severe opportunistic infections and probable chances of developing malignancy [5–9]. Transplant recipients are having increased chances of developing cancers and high mortality and morbidity rate. The main key point here is that immunosuppressive treatment procures the complications. However, if there is a reduction in immunosuppressive therapy, it can lead to rejection of the graft. The associated evaluating factors like biochemical, microbiological, and imaging parameters are not always sufficient for diagnosis. The role of FDG PET-CT is to detect metabolic changes seen in malignant and inflammatory cells and is most widely used to localize, stage, and monitor response to treatment of their respective pathologies. In one of the studies at Copen Hagen University Hospital, the database of management of posttransplant infections in collaborating hospitals (MATCH) program the impact of post transplant complications was studied. This was one of the pioneering studies involving liver, lung, kidney, and heart transplantations in Denmark. FDG PET-CT was performed in these patients to evaluate the underlying infective focus after the transplantation and to follow up for any progression of transplant rejection. This quantification of FDG PET-CT whole-body scan was based on normal infection, malignancy, inconclusive and/or other clinical details. The results of FDG PET-CT were compared with the final clinical diagnosis by two independent physicians and classified as true-positive, true-negative, false-positive, false-negative contributory to diagnosis, contributory to exclusion, noncontributory. In one of the studies, with 1814 solid organ transplant recipients, 219 FDG PET-CT scans were performed. Of this, 122 (84% recipients) were not diagnosed by FDG PET-CT and 133 scans were done under this indication. The evaluation was done with associated fever of unknown origin protocol, where organ-specific symptoms like diarrhea, stomach pain, coughing, and neurological symptoms were documented. The other aspect of evaluation is by altered biochemical or microbial markers like CRP, LDH, ALT, or PCR (polymerase chain reaction). The final diagnosis in relation to FDG PET-CT ($N = 133$) by done by evalauting these various parameters. The diagnostic workup shows cancers, and infections as the commonest causes of rejection. The diagnostic value of FDG PET in these patients shows significant sensitivity, specificity, positive predictive, and negative predictive values of 97, 84, 87, and 96%, respectively. Here the correlation with the symptoms and the amount of probable rejection activity is not correlating with the FDG PET-CT findings. However, FDG PET is sensitive for evaluating the cause of rejection and associated information or findings predisposing the rejection. FUO (fever of unknown origin) protocol is followed here especially in relation to the evaluation of infective focus than the extent of involvement.

FDG PET-CT is the noninvasive imaging tool for the evaluation of any pathology based on the amount of glycolytic activity. In this process, the activated inflammatory cells like neutrophils, macrophages, and lymphocytes cause increased uptake.

19.3 FDG Analysis

The FDG PET-CT is an important modality that contributes to a lot of diagnostic information:

1. Identifying the site of the infection
2. Rule out the malignancy
3. Extent of the infection and organs involved
4. Targeting the diagnostic procedure
5. Follow-up of the infection after treatment

19.4 Liver Transplantation

Liver transplantation is commonly advised in the cases of hepatic failure which is end-stage chronic liver disease. One of another commonest causes of liver transplantation is in HCC (hepatocellular carcinoma). The HCC is one of the six most common causes of cancer due to associated risk of hepatitis-B and hepatitis-C virus infection. One of the predisposing factors is nonalcoholic fatty liver disease. Thus, there is a strong link between cirrhosis and HCC. One of the important entities in transplantation is the vascular invasion which is an important predictor of recurrence and ultimate survival of transplant. As per Toronto criteria which is histological criteria this asscoiated infections related to post transplant HCC were studied. The transplant tumor biopsy is not done commonly. The sensitivity of biopsy depends on the location of the tumor, needle size, and tumor size. Alpha Feto protein is one of the important reference biomarkers of HCC. Immediate posttransplant liver imaging usually is to be done ideally around 6 weeks. If done prior, there is a high chance of false-positive information due to postoperative changes. However, with the advent of PET, the associated infection in the transplanted organ has high sensitivity for PET-CT [9–13]. SUV values thus play an important role in the management of various tumor markers.

FDG PET-CT in the evaluation of posttransplant has detection rates of 100% and size is also one of the important criteria. One of the graft posttransplant rejection secondary to infection shows diffuse increased uptake which is consistent with infective focus. Other parameters of diffuse posttransplant hepatic infections show diffuse increased uptake in liver parenchyma, focal uptake, perihepatic collection, perihepatic fat stranding/peritoneal stranding, and inflammatory changes in the porta at the site of graft [14–18]. Thus, FDG uptake can characterize the direct and indirect findings of hepatic failure after liver transplantation (Figs. 19.1, 19.2 and 19.3).

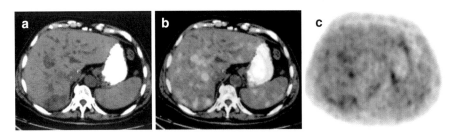

Fig. 19.1 Post-liver transplant PET-CT at the level of the liver. CT image (**a**) showing irregular hypodensities in the right lobe. Fused and PET images (**b** and **c**) showing mild uptake in this hypodense lesion with SUV max of 7.1 suggestive of posttransplant infection

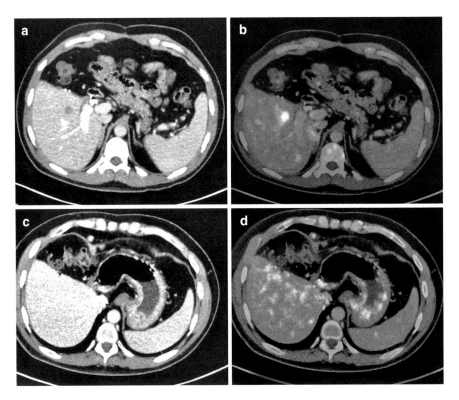

Fig. 19.2 Post-liver transplant PET-CT at the level of liver showing small hypodense lesion on CT image (**a**) in segment-V with significant tracer activity. SUV max of 6.5 fused image (**b**) suggestive of posttransplant infection. Image courtesy Dr. Suneetha Batchu, Asian Institute of Gastroenterology, Hyderabad

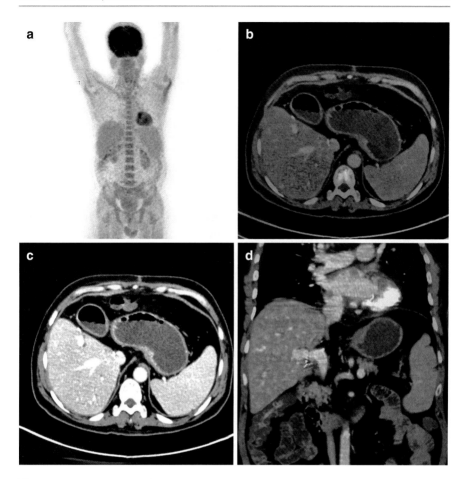

Fig. 19.3 Whole-body post-liver transplant PET-CT. CT, image (**c**), PET image (**a**) and fused images (**b**, **d**) showing no abnormal metabolic activity focus suggestive of no abnormality. Image courtesy Dr. Suneetha Batchu, Asian Institute of Gastroenterology, Hyderabad

19.5   Renal Transplantation

Renal transplant is one of the important lines of management in chronic renal diseases with significantly elevated serum creatinine. The role of FDG PET-CT is the same. The criterion for evaluation remains the same as 6 weeks. However, the early transplant rejection also shows equivocal findings of that of postoperative changes. Here, FDG PET-CT findings have to be correlated with the associated parameters like serum creatinine of perinephric collections by imaging, cortex and medullary differentiation and associated Doppler findings. Any doubtful case to be differentiated between the transplant rejection any associated underlying pathology FDG PET has plays an important role. The findings in PET-CT are increased attenuation of kidneys, cortical irregularity,

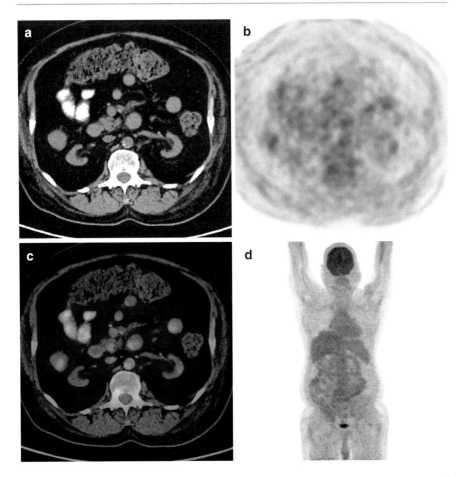

Fig. 19.4 Whole-body PET-CT renal failure patient. CT image (**a**) showing bilateral contracted small-sized kidneys with no abnormal metabolic activity in fused image (**c**) and PET images (**b, d**)

perinephric fat stranding, and perinephric collections. In the early phases of posttransplantation, PET-CT findings have to be correlated with other lab findings [24, 25] (Figs. 19.4 and 19.5).

19.6 Cardiac Transplantation

Cardiac transplantation is one of the common entities, usually done in end-stage heart failure disease. The PET-CT criterion remains the same. The amount of uptake in the evaluation of FDG PET-CT is not common. However, due to the vitality of the heart, the transplantation is the mainstay treatment especially in associated background findings also. The transplant rejection findings for cardiac are not well established. However, with this advent of challenging aspects of the cardiac transplantation expertise use and other findings in the evaluation of PET-CT after

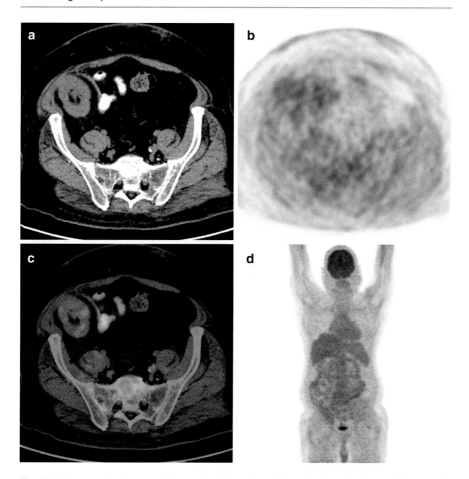

Fig. 19.5 Same patient post-renal transplant. Transplant kidney in right iliac fossa CT image (**a**) showing no abnormal metabolic activity in fused image (**c**) and PET images (**b**, **d**) consistent with no posttransplant complications

cardiac transplantation is challenging. The FDG PET in the commonly used. However, ammonia cardiac scan is also being used for evaluation. The protocol followed is of fever of unknown origin. Here the differentiation has to be made with other underlying/associated causes like tuberculosis or any associated infections or any associated cardiac pathology involving pericardium, epicardium, myocardium and endocardium [26, 29].

19.7 Lung Transplantation

Lung transplantation is rare entity done worldwide. However, our Yashoda group of Hospitals is privileged to have done first successful lung transplantation. The evaluation of this transplant organ is also based on the same criteria of liver/kidney transplantations. The rejection pattern in lung transplantation is not well established due to very few lung transplants and that two very few PET scans evaluation after the transplantation [30, 31].

Heart–lung transplantation is also done concurrently because of concurrent pathology involved.

19.8   Posttransplant Lymphoproliferative Disorders

Posttransplant lymphoproliferative disorders are important heterogeneous group of disorders occurring commonly after solid organ transplant or Allogeneic hematopoietic cell transplant. As per the WHO classification this PTLD is classified as early lesion PTLD (non-destructive), monomorphic PTLD (B-cell, T-cell NK-cell), polymorphic PTLD and Hodgkin's lymphoma PTLD [32]. PTLDs are serious posttransplant complications with significant morbidity and mortality [19–22]. So accurate diagnosis and timely diagnosis is important. The role of FDG PET-CT in the initial work up of PTLD is defined by the guidelines from the American Society of Transplantation. Here the information for staging and treatment response is done by FDG PET. In one of the studies by Montes De Jeses et al. [23] retrospective study in evaluation of suspected PTLD. FDG PET-CT sensitivity, specificity, positive and negative predictive values, and accuracies were 85%, 90%, 83%, 92% and 89% respectively. These results show excellent diagnostic performance by FDG PET-CT in detecting PTLD. With few false-positive PTLD results by FDG PET-CT still the FDG PET-CT is clinically relevant.

19.9   Conclusion

FDG PET-CT is emerging modality for diagnosis, staging and treatment response assessment in various heterogeneous pattern of patients in various organ transplantation and in PTLD.

FDG PET-CT is important modality for the evaluation of unexplained inflammatory syndrome, FUO and other dormant lesion which becomes active.

The comparative analysis with different imaging modalities in pediatric and adult patients FDG PET-CT is important modality. However, PET-MRI has become a particularly good alternative because of no ionizing radiation and high soft tissue sensitivity in picking up very small subtle lesions.

References

1. Lin CY, Liao CW, Chu LY, Yen KY, Jeng LB, Hsu CN, Lin CL, Kao CH. Predictive value of 18F-FDG PET/CT for vascular invasion in patients with hepatocellular carcinoma before liver transplantation. Clin Nucl Med. 2017;42:e183–7. https://doi.org/10.1097/RLU.0000000000001545.

2. Denton MD, Magee CC, Sayegh MH. Immunosuppressive strategies in transplantation. Lancet. 1999;353(9158):1083–91.
3. Apel H, Walschburger-Zorn K, Haberle L, Wach S, Engehausen DG, Wullich B. De novo malignancies in renal transplant recipients: experience at a single center with 1882 transplant patients over 39 yr. Clin Transpl. 2013;27(1):E30–6.
4. Guba M, Graeb C, Jauch KW, Geissler EK. Pro- and anti-cancer effects of immunosuppressive agents used in organ transplantation. Transplantation. 2004;77(12):1777–82.
5. Li J, Liu Y, Wang Z. Multimodality imaging features, treatment, and prognosis of post-transplant lymphoproliferative disorder in renal allografts. Medicine (Baltimore). 2018;97(17):e0531.
6. Acuna SA, Huang JW, Daly C, Shah PS, Kim SJ, Baxter NN. Outcomes of solid organ transplant recipients with preexisting malignancies in remission: a systematic review and meta-analysis. Transplantation. 2017;101(3):471–81.
7. Al-Mansour Z, Nelson BP, Evens AM. Post-transplant lymphoproliferative disease (PTLD): risk factors, diagnosis, and current treatment strategies. Curr Hematol Malig Rep. 2013;8(3):173–83.
8. Schlansky B, Chen Y, Scott DL, Austin D, Naughler WE. Waiting time predicts survival after liver transplantation for hepatocellular carcinoma: a cohort study using the united network for organ sharing registry. Liver Transpl. 2014;20:1045–56.
9. Hong G, Suh KS, Suh SW, Yoo T, Kim H, Park MS, Choi Y, Paeng JC, Yi NJ, Lee KW. Alpha-fetoprotein and (18)F-FDG positron emission tomography predict tumor recurrence better than Milan criteria in living donor liver transplantation. J Hepatol. 2016;64:852–9. https://doi.org/10.1016/j.jhep.2015.11.033.
10. McGlynn KA, London WT. The global epidemiology of hepatocellular carcinoma: present and future. Clin Liver Dis. 2011;15:223–43, vii–vix. https://doi.org/10.1016/j.cld.2011.03.006
11. Yang JD, Larson JJ, Watt KD, Allen AM, Wiesner RH, Gores GJ, Roberts LR, Heimbach JA, Leise MD. Hepatocellular carcinoma is the most common indication for liver transplantation and placement on the waitlist in the United States. Clin Gastroenterol Hepatol. 2017;15:767–775.e3. https://doi.org/10.1016/j.cgh.2016.11.034.
12. Mazzaferro V, Regalia E, Doci R, Andreola S, Pulvirenti A, Bozzetti F, Montalto F, Ammatuna M, Morabito A, Gennari L. Liver transplantation for the treatment of small hepatocellular carcinomas in patients with cirrhosis. N Engl J Med. 1996;334:693–9. https://doi.org/10.1056/NEJM199603143341104].
13. Yao FY, Ferrell L, Bass NM, Watson JJ, Bacchetti P, Venook A, Ascher NL, Roberts JP. Liver transplantation for hepatocellular carcinoma: expansion of the tumor size limits does not adversely impact survival. Hepatology. 2001;33:1394–403. https://doi.org/10.1053/jhep.2001.24563].
14. Sotiropoulos GC, Malagó M, Molmenti E, Paul A, Nadalin S, Brokalaki E, Kühl H, Dirsch O, Lang H, Broelsch CE. Liver transplantation for hepatocellular carcinoma in cirrhosis: is clinical tumor classification before transplantation realistic? Transplantation. 2005;79:483–7. https://doi.org/10.1097/01.TP.0000152801.82734.74.
15. Hemming AW, Cattral MS, Reed AI, Van Der Werf WJ, Greig PD, Howard RJ. Liver transplantation for hepatocellular carcinoma. Ann Surg. 2001;233:652–9. https://doi.org/10.1097/00000658-200105000-00009.
16. Roayaie S, Schwartz JD, Sung MW, Emre SH, Miller CM, Gondolesi GE, Krieger NR, Schwartz ME. Recurrence of hepatocellular carcinoma after liver transplant: patterns and prognosis. Liver Transpl. 2004;10:534–40. https://doi.org/10.1002/lt.20128.
17. Shirabe K, Itoh S, Yoshizumi T, Soejima Y, Taketomi A, Aishima S, Maehara Y. The predictors of microvascular invasion in candidates WJGO. www.wjgnet.com. October 15, 2018; 10(10) (Yaprak O et al. Role of 18F-FDG PET/CT in LT for HCC. 50:682–687. https://doi.org/10.2967/jnumed.108.060574)
18. Fishman JA. Infection in solid-organ transplant recipients. N Engl J Med. 2007;357(25):2601–14.
19. Bakker NA, van Imhoff GW, Verschuuren EA, van Son WJ. Presentation and early detection of post-transplant lymphoproliferative disorder after solid organ transplantation. Transpl Int. 2007;20(3):207–18.

20. Blaes AH, Cioc AM, Froelich JW, Peterson BA, Dunitz JM. Positron emission tomography scanning in the setting of post transplant lympho-proliferative disorders. Clin Transpl. 2009;23(6):794–9.
21. Van Keerberghen CA, Goffin K, Vergote V, Tousseyn T, Verhoef G, Laenen A, et al. Role of interim and end of treatment positron emission tomography for response assessment and prediction of relapse in post transplant lympho-proliferative disorder. Acta Oncol. 2019;58(7):1041–7.
22. Zimmermann H, Denecke T, Dreyling MH, Franzius C, Reinke P, Subklewe M, et al. End-of-treatment positron emission tomography after uniform first-line therapy of B-cell post transplant lympho-proliferative disorder identifies patients at low risk of relapse in the prospective German PTLD registry. Transplantation. 2018;102(5):868–75.
23. Montes de Jesus FM, Kwee TC, Nijland M, Kahle XU, Huls G, Dierckx RAJO, et al. Performance of advanced imaging modalities at diagnosis and treatment response evaluation of patients with post-transplant lymphoproliferative disorder: a systematic review and meta-analysis. Crit Rev Oncol Hematol. 2018;132(June):27–38.
24. Stallone G, Infante B, Grandaliano G, et al. Management and prevention of post-transplant malignancies in kidney transplant recipients. Clin Kidney J. 2015;8(5):637–44.
25. Jadoul A, Lovinfosse P, Bouquegneau A, et al. Observer variability in the assessment of renal ^{18}F-FDG uptake in kidney transplant recipients. Sci Rep. 2020;10:4617.
26. Muller N, Kessler R, Caillard S, Epailly E, Hubelé F, Heimburger C, et al. (18)F-FDG PET/CT for the diagnosis of malignant and infectious complications after solid organ transplantation. Nucl Med Mol Imaging. 2017;51(1):58–68.
27. Rechavia E, de Silva R, Kushwaha SS, et al. Enhanced myocardial 18F-2-fluoro-2-deoxyglucose uptake after orthotopic heart transplantation assessed by positron emission tomography. J Am Coll Cardiol. 1997;30(2):533.
28. Dandel M, Hetzer R. Post-transplant surveillance for acute rejection and allograft vasculopathy by echocardiography: usefulness of myocardial velocity and deformation imaging. J Heart Lung Transplant. 2017;36:117–31.
29. Lund LH, Khush KK, Cherikh WS, et al. The registry of the International Society for Heart and Lung Transplantation: thirty-fourth adult heart transplantation report—2017; focus theme: allograft ischemic time. J Heart Lung Transplant. 2017;36:1037–46.
30. Chambers DC, Cherikh WS, Goldfarb SB, et al. The international thoracic organ transplant registry of the International Society for Heart and Lung Transplantation: thirty-fifth adult lung and heart-lung transplant report-2018; focus theme: multiorgan transplantation. J Heart Lung Transplant. 2018;37(10):1169–83.
31. Yusen RD, Edwards LB, Kucheryavaya AY, et al. The registry of the International Society for Heart and Lung Transplantation: thirty-second official adult lung and heart-lung transplantation report—2015; focus theme: early graft failure. J Heart Lung Transplant. 2015;34(10):1264–77.
32. Wolfe CR, Ison MG. AST infectious diseases community of practice. Donor-derived infections: guidelines from the American Society of Transplantation infectious diseases Community of Practice. Clin Transpl. 2019;33(9):e13547.

Molecular Imaging in Infection and Inflammation

20

Key Points

Molecular imaging or functional imaging is an imaging at the cellular level which can improve the diagnosis of the diseases at an earlier stage. This includes many pathologies like malignancies, atherosclerosis, infection, inflammation, and other research areas. In this, the quantification of the disease pathophysiology can be done which acts like biomarkers of inflammation, thus helping to diagnose disease, establish the prognosis, and respond to the preventive and therapeutic options.

20.1 Introduction

Molecular imaging is the noninvasive imaging of cellular and subcellular level [1]. Molecular imaging is rapidly developing imaging modality with the concept of personalized medicine [2, 3]. Molecular imaging has got more importance in recent years due to the significant depth and breadth as a research and clinical discipline. This is possible with the combination with the advances in engineering, molecular biology, chemistry, immunology, and genetics and combined with the multi- and interdisciplinary innovations. This is leading to the many newer concepts of clinical noninvasive imaging strategies which lead to better disease identification, risk stratification, and monitoring of therapy effects with remarkably high sensitivity and specificity. This will have a significant impact on the treatment regimens and influence of the various parameters.

Molecular imaging is the advanced version of functional imaging modalities like FDG PET-CT. It offers unique and unsurpassed possibilities for better evaluation of various pathologies. Infective inflammatory pathologies are the recent developments in this molecular imaging modality. The common questions which are answered are infective focus, inflammatory sign, the extent of the lesion, involvement of the various organs, therapeutic options, monitoring response to treatment, and potential

© The Author(s), under exclusive license to Springer Nature
Singapore Pte Ltd. 2021
S. Shaikh, *PET-CT in Infection and Inflammation*,
https://doi.org/10.1007/978-981-15-9801-2_20

impacts of the side effects on the patient. Till now, hybrid imaging modality FDG PET-CT was commonly used and being used worldwide for evaluation of infection and inflammation [4, 5]. Till date, the nuclear medicine imaging techniques like positron emission tomography (PET), PET combined with computed tomography (CT), and single-photon emission computed tomography were the most widely used imaging modalities. However, now due to advancements in various imaging techniques in magnetic resonance (MR), optical, CT, and ultrasonographic (US) imaging, these imaging techniques are widely being used in the future. CT uses the X-ray attenuation so cannot be used as the imaging modality of Molecular Imaging.

20.2   Pathophysiology

The basis of inflammation is the accumulation of fluid in extracellular space, endothelial disruption, and organ damage. The accumulation of leukocytes macrophages, monocytes, lymphocytes, and giant cells constitute the body's response to injury and infection [6]. With this, the response of the immune system is the activation of the pro- and anti-inflammatory secretions like cytokine, chemokines. After this, another important modality PET-MR is also now commonly used, especially in the borderline conditions were subtle findings are missed by the PET-CT. Few of the examples are sarcoidosis, osteomyelitis, spinal infection, fever of unknown origin, metastatic infection, bacteremia, and vasculitis [7]. But despite these applications, there are subtle imaging findings which cannot be evaluated by these hybrid imaging modalities. Certain infections like fungal, vascular graft, joint prosthesis, infections in diabetes, endocarditis, inflammatory bowel diseases, and infective inflammatory diseases occur in the pediatric age group.

20.3   Imaging of Macrophages and Monocytes

In any infection and inflammation, macrophages and monocytes are important. This has been important in the setting of inflammation [8, 9]. The imaging of these cells can be done by using small and ultra-small paramagnetic iron oxide nanoparticles SPIO and USPIO [10, 11]. The basis of this uptake is the phagocytosis. This evaluation can be done on the characteristic features of surface coating and opsonization. There are a couple of factors for the modification depending on the size, surface coating, and adding specific ligands with an impact on the amount of the uptake. Macrophages can also be imaged by using the PET and SPECT ligands and optical imaging.

20.4   Imaging of Lymphocytes

B lymphocytes are the important components of the hormonal immunity component and adaptive immune system by the production of various antibodies in response to various antigens. The various subtypes of the B cells are also identified by various

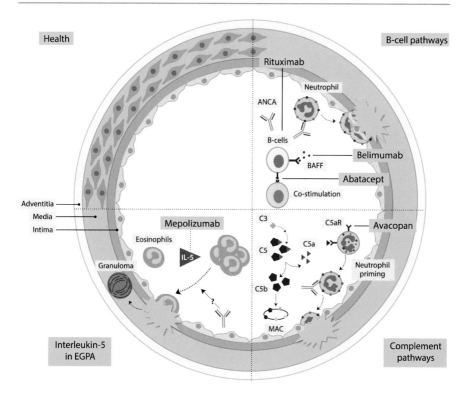

Fig. 20.1   Molecular imaging of various mechanisms and pathways

cell markers. The B cell function and dysfunction can lead to various autoimmune diseases making these pathogenic B cells the main components of this process. Rituximab is the radiolabeled marker used in patients with rheumatoid arthritis, psoriatic arthritis, and sarcoidosis. Radio-immunotherapy's response also plays an important role [12, 13].

T cell lymphocytes are important in cell-mediated immune response. Imaging of this T lymphocytes is important for detecting the inflammation and autoimmune disorders. Many radiotracers are being used to identify the various applications. Radiolabeled cytokines are also used [14] (Fig. 20.1).

20.5   Imaging of Inflammation at the Organ Level

20.5.1   Central Nervous System Inflammation

Neuroinflammation is suspected in various infections like HIV, neurodegenerative diseases, brain tumors, and psychiatric diseases. The most common protocol in the neuroinflammation imaging is through targeting the translocator protein, mitochondrial membrane receptor that becomes upregulated in activated microglia, astrocytes, and blood-derived macrophages in the central nervous system. Other potential targets for neuroinflammation imaging are being used now [15]. Neuroinflammatory changes can be evaluated with targeted iron oxide magnetic nanoparticles for the evaluation of infarct. In certain conditions like multiple sclerosis, magnetic nanoparticles are more specific than gadolinium [16].

20.5.2 Vascular Diseases and Atherosclerosis

Imaging of atherosclerosis is of more interest due to the inflammation macrophage activity and the risk of plaque development and rupture. 18 F FDG is well established for the evaluation of inflammatory vascular plaques and corresponds with the macrophage activity [17]. TSPO expression and radiolabeled DOTATATE acts in various cell populations [18]. SPIO nanoparticles are also used in atherosclerosis (Fig. 20.2).

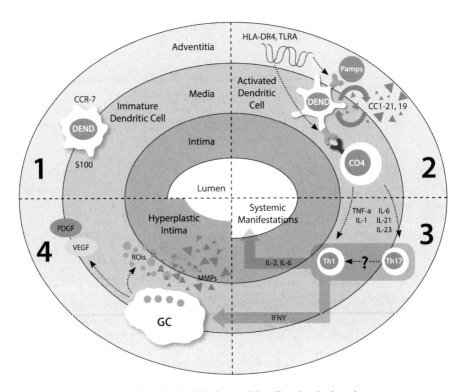

Fig. 20.2 Various mechanisms involved in the arterial wall molecular imaging processes

20.5.3 Chest, Abdominal Organs and Joints

Imaging of the inflammation in the lungs [19, 20] and various abdominal organs is well established. 18 F FDG PET is found to be useful in post-radiation pneumonitis, cystic fibrosis, and asthma.

In myocardial infarction, the accumulation of USPIOs over time suggests inflammatory cells [21]. This however is of not much clinical relevance. 18 F FDG PET is well established in peripheral inflammatory arthritis [22, 23]. Another aspect is the usefulness of 18 F FDG PET and USPIO in the settings of Systemic Lupus Erythematosus and Sjogren Syndrome.

20.5.4 Optical Imaging

In optical imaging process, fluorophores are used to generate an optical signal on excitation by an external light source of a specific wavelength [24]. Indocyanine green can be used are the fluorophore which can be conjugated to a targeting molecule for evaluating the image specific areas of interest. The emitted signal is captured by a sensitive charge-coupled device camera. The biggest advantage of optical imaging is to evaluate fast imaging with high-resolution images. The advantage of the optical imaging is that it does not require radioactivity, is cheaper and more flexible than radionuclide imaging, and can be repeated without ionization of the molecules. The disadvantage is the fluorescence signal can penetrate up to a maximum depth of only 1 cm. Thus, optical imaging is mainly for superficial imaging.

The newer imaging technique of optoacoustic is photoacoustic imaging which has a more penetration depth and the scan evaluates more potential clinical applications [25, 26].

Optoacoustic imaging is based on thermal expansion of a tissue of interest which is caused by short laser pulses by intrinsic fluorophores [27]. Here focused detectors register ultrasonic fissure waves generated through thermoelastic expansion of the fluorophores. The penetration here is 3–5 cm approximately. With this, the field of molecular optical and optoacoustic imaging [28] is rapidly evolving with close synergy with modalities like PET, SPECT, MR, and ultrasound. With the advent of PET-MR, the two separate modalities allow tissue characterization and physiological localization better by PET signals within the soft tissues [29]. PET-MR has an advantage in conditions like insulitis, spondylodiscitis, inflammatory bowel disease, soft tissue infection, neurological infection, and inflammation. Molecular ultrasound is based on the diagnostic and therapeutic ultrasound [30]. Therapeutic ultrasound is used mostly for thermal or mechanical effects. The non-thermal ultrasound energy is used for combination treatment with drugs for various diseases [31]. With the development of microbubbles, molecular targeted agents and carriers or enhancers of drug this imaging modality is becoming more precise and specific [32]. The role of ultrasound after irradiation of tissues and cells enhancing drug target is also becoming more important. Efficient delivery of the drugs into target cells or tissues is a challenge.

20.5.5 Ultrasound Molecular Imaging

Molecular ultrasound imaging is now an important component of the molecular imaging. The biggest advantage is the noninvasive nature and no radiation makes this modality of choice for various applications. With the fast development of molecular biology and ultrasound contrast agents ultrasound as a modality is redefined due to its molecular imaging applications. Ultrasound can detect changes in the molecular markers on the vascular endothelium and other intravascular targets. This new concept is referred to as ultrasonic molecular imaging. In many studies, ultrasonic molecular imaging has shown an important role in assessing angiogenesis, inflammation, and thrombus. Microbubble contrast agents with ultrasound technology, and signal processing strategies have the potential to substantially improve the capabilities and utility of ultrasonic molecular imaging [33, 34].

20.5.6 MR Molecular Imaging

MRI as an imaging modality has excellent soft-tissue resolution and gives excellent information about the tissue architecture. It is a modality that has no radiation. The targeted agents used in MRI-based molecular imaging are not as sensitive as that of agents used in PET and SPECT due to its little bigger size.

MRI-based detection of inflammation is done after injection of the contrast agents which can cause nonspecific changes in inflamed tissues as magnetic nanoparticles as MRI contrast agents with their ability to disturb the relaxation of nearby protons can be detected by MRI. Nanoparticles can be used to detect vascular leak and this principle can detect pancreatic inflammation in patients with type 1 diabetes. Nanoparticles are phagocytosed by macrophages, so IO-containing formulations cause a darkening of the reticuloendothelial system in the liver and spleen on T_2-weighted images. Darkening of tissues by IO nanoparticles can therefore be employed as a marker of inflammation. This approach has also been used to detect inflammation in patients with renal transplant rejection, atherosclerosis, and multiple sclerosis [35–40].

Noninvasive detection of endothelial inflammation with MRI and VCAM-1 or P-selectin-targeted MPIO was possible in atherosclerosis, unilateral ischemia/reperfusion injury of kidneys, and cerebral ischemia, focal brain ischemia, blood–brain barrier breakdown, and brain inflammation were noninvasively detected with MRI and E- and P-selectin-targeted gadolinium diethylenetriaminepentaacetic acid (Gd-DTPA) conjugated with E- and P-selectin-binding Sialyl Lewis carbohydrate antigen.

Thus, the detection of tissue inflammation using MRI-based molecular imaging in diseases is important as detailed anatomic information regarding the localization of the target molecule is critical to the diagnosis.

20.5.7 Nanoimaging

Nanoimaging is the important evolving molecular imaging technique that is being widely used using the various nanoparticle contrast agents for evaluation of various pathologies. The molecular imaging probes are used in this process, and with the technological advancements, the probe design is increased significantly. The probe design used here is to detect the multifunctionality, more efficient targeting, better biocompatibility, and agents. The ideal nanoparticles used in imaging should have specific formulations for easy use and it depends on many factors like their biocompatibility, efficacy, specificity, and detection of further disease targets.

There are many nanoparticles which are used for nanotechnology applications in cancer therapeutics and imaging. Carbon nanotubes are made up of the sheets of carbon atoms that are one-atom thick and that are rolled into a seamless cylindrical carbon molecule and these are widely used to detect and image DNA mutations and proteins and have been found to generate lethal heat when exposed to radiofrequency fields. Dendrimers are repeatedly branched molecules. Folic acid, gold nanoparticles, and chemotherapeutics are mixed with dendrimers, thus allowing them a large number of imaging or therapeutic moieties on the surface of the tumor cell. These dendromeric agents are used for controlled drug release and photodynamic-thermal therapy as well as contrast agents for all imaging modalities. Functional contrast agents such as gadolinium and radionuclides, chemotherapeutics, photodynamic therapeutics, and reactive oxygen species are also used for targeted imaging or therapy.

Thus, nanoparticles can be made multifunctional by linking it with functional moieties for imaging, targeting, stabilizing, and therapeutic functional groups have been described. Radiolabeled antibodies, antibody Fab fragments, and ligands have been used in nuclear medicine for imaging and treatment for decades.

SPIO is being widely used for the inflammatory or degenerative diseases, and also for the imaging of stem cell migration and immune cell trafficking. The iodinated, bismuth, and gold nanoparticle-based CT contrast agents are also being developed which can be used in the CT scan. Nanoparticles are also used in the construction of the reporter moieties to detect intracellular processes such as apoptosis and synthesis of particular proteins; this will be useful for molecular imaging. Novel nanoparticle-based therapeutics can be used for pain control with transdermal local anesthetics, sustained-release antimicrobials for treatment of infection. The use of nano-capsules and liposomes as hemoglobin carriers are being developed as blood substitutes. Drug-eluting stents which release agents such as sirolimus and paclitaxel are having the potential to reduce intimal hyperplasia that can prevent restenosis.

Interventional molecular imaging helps in the minimally invasive procedures like (e.g., percutaneous, catheter-directed intravascular, and endoluminal) placement of imaging tools, such as optical imaging probes. With this, the applications of molecular imaging techniques are to reach deep-seated targets, enable a close look at small targets, precisely guiding the delivery of non-targeted imaging tracers or therapeutic agents, and super selectively enhance the effectiveness of targeted imaging [41–47].

The last resort will be the imaging of the therapeutic response of various conditions where nanoparticles are used. With this, the evaluation can be analyzed before the anatomical changes.

20.5.8 Limitations of Molecular Imaging

The limitations of the hybrid imaging modalities are not clear delineation of infection from sterile inflammation, malignancy, and physiological wound healing. For this sort of condition, more specific targeted radiopharmaceuticals and imaging techniques are needed. One of the classic applications is labeled white blood cells which is specific for infection and used commonly to evaluate osteomyelitis, joint prosthesis, and diabetic foot infections. One of the important radiopharmaceuticals is ^{99m}Tc-labeled interleukin-2 which is specific for interleukin-2 receptors. This process is overexpressed by activated T lymphocytes during inflammation.

A couple of agents where molecular imaging is used are humanized antibodies such as bevacizumab or trastuzumab. One of the infection-specific imaging tracers is antibiotic ciprofloxacin which was labeled with ^{99m}Tc and 18F to specifically target bacteria. The challenging concept here is to distinguish inflammation from infection but also to determine positive microorganism. One of the common examples is *streptococcus pyogenes* in necrotizing fasciitis is of help in evaluating whether the surgical procedure is needed or not. Similarly, other organisms also can be evaluated by this process.

Thus, molecular imaging is not limited to radionuclide [48, 49] but also can be performed by optical imaging.

20.6   Conclusion

With the advancement in techniques and translational medicine, molecular imaging has evolved as a new diagnostic era. Oncology is most commonly used for molecular imaging. Common pathology is infectious and inflammatory diseases and thus the combination of molecular imaging techniques can clearly categorize the pathophysiological processes and pathogens involved at highlighting the cells, potential target for evaluating the pathogenic bacteria and biological active molecules for both diagnosis and treatment options. More targets and corresponding ligands within the immune system and various organs can be evaluated better. With this, probably in the future, it will be the era of personalized medicine.

With the Nanotechnology, Nanoimaging, has evolved into the important diagnostic and therapeutic imaging modalities more commonly used for evaluation of molecular diagnosis. It has a diagnostic and therapeutic component. Diagnostic is for diagnosis and therapeutic is a treatment option. Most of these imaging modalities are using nanoparticles like nanopores. Like this, the nanoparticles are also used in therapeutic options.

References

1. David A, Mankoff A. Definition of molecular imaging. J Nucl Med. 2007;48:18N–21N.
2. Signore A, Erba PA. Editorial: molecular imaging of inflammation/infection: the future of disease management. Curr Pharm Des. 2018;24(7):741–2.
3. Signore A, Anzola KL, Auletta S, Varani M, Petitti A, Pacilio M, Galli F, Lauri C. Current status of molecular imaging in inflammatory and autoimmune disorders. Curr Pharm Des. 2018;24(7):743–53.
4. Ametamey SM, Honer M, Schubiger PA. Molecular imaging with PET. Chem Rev. 2008;108(5):1501–16.
5. Heneweer C, Grimm J. Clinical applications in molecular imaging. Pediatr Radiol. 2011;41(2):199–207.
6. Liu Y, Ghesani NV, Zuckier LS. Physiology and pathophysiology of incidental findings detected on FDG-PET scintigraphy. Semin Nucl Med. 2010;40:294–315.
7. Jung K-H, Lee K-H. Molecular imaging in the era of personalized medicine. J Pathol Transl Med. 2015;49(1):5–12.
8. Kubota R, Yamada S, Kubota K, Ishiwata K, Tamahashi N, Ido T. Intratumoral distribution of fluorine-18-fluorodeoxyglucose in vivo: high accumulation in macrophages and granulation tissues studied by microautoradiography. J Nucl Med. 1992;33:1972–80.
9. Rua R, McGavern DB. Elucidation of monocyte/macrophage dynamics and function by intravital imaging. J Leukoc Biol. 2015;98:319–32.
10. Nighoghossian N, Wiart M, Cakmak S, et al. Inflammatory response after ischemic stroke: a USPIO-enhanced MRI study in patients. Stroke. 2007;38:303–7.
11. Taupitz SPIOM, Schmitz S, Hamm B. Super-paramagnetic iron oxide particles: current state and future development. Rofo. 2003;175(6):752–65.
12. Malviya G, Anzola KL, Podesta E, et al. ^{99m}Tc-labeled rituximab for imaging B lymphocyte infiltration in inflammatory autoimmune disease patients. Mol Imaging Biol. 2012;14:637–46.
13. Iodice V, Laganà B, Lauri C, et al. Imaging B lymphocytes in autoimmune inflammatory diseases. Q J Nucl Med Mol Imaging. 2014;58(3):258–68.
14. MacIver NJ, Michalek RD, Rathmell JC. Metabolic regulation of T lymphocytes. Annu Rev Immunol. 2013;31:259–83.
15. Neuwelt A, Sidhu N, Hu CA, Mlady G, Eberhardt SC, Sillerud LO. Iron-based super-paramagnetic nanoparticle contrast agents for MRI of infection and inflammation. AJR. 2015;204:W302–13.
16. Savonenko AV, Melnikova T, Wang Y, et al. Cannabinoid CB2 receptors in a mouse model of Abeta amyloidosis: immune-histochemical analysis and suitability as a PET biomarker of neuro-inflammation. PLoS One. 2015;10:e0129618.
17. Bala G, Blykers A, Xavier C, et al. Targeting of vascular cell adhesion molecule-1 by ^{18}F-labelled nanobodies for PET/CT imaging of inflamed atherosclerotic plaque. Eur Heart J Cardiovasc Imaging. 2016. 22; Epub ahead of print.
18. Owen DR, Yeo AJ, Gunn RN, et al. An 18-kDa translocator protein (TSPO) polymorphism explains differences in binding affinity of the PET radioligand PBR28. J Cereb Blood Flow Metab. 2012;32:1–5.
19. Prager E, Wehrschuetz M, Bisail B, et al. Comparison of 18F-FDG and 67Gacitrate in sarcoidosis imaging. Nuklearmedizin. 2008;47:18–23.
20. Anderson CJ, Lewis JS. Current status and future challenges for molecular imaging. Philos Trans A Math Phys Eng Sci. 2017;375:20170023. https://doi.org/10.1098/rsta.2017.0023.
21. Storey P, Lim RP, Chandarana H, et al. MRI assessment of hepatic iron clearance rates after USPIO administration in healthy adults. Investig Radiol. 2012;47(12):717–24.
22. Biswal S, Resnick DL, Hoffman JM, Gambhir SS. Molecular imaging: integration of molecular imaging into the musculoskeletal imaging practice. Radiology. 2007;244:651–71.

23. Bar I, Zilberman Y, Zeira E, et al. Molecular imaging of the skeleton: quantitative real time bioluminescence monitoring gene expression in bone repair and development. J Bone Miner Res. 2003;18:570–8.
24. Rabe J-H, Sammour DA, Schulz S, Munteanu B, Ott M, Ochs K, Hohenberger P, Marx A, Platten M, Opitz C, et al. Fourier transform infrared microscopy enables guidance of automated mass spectrometry imaging to predefined tissue morphologies. Sci Rep. 2018.
25. Branchini BR, Ablamsky DM, Davis AL, Southworth TL, Butler B, Fan F, et al. Red-emitting luciferases for bioluminescence reporter and imaging applications. Anal Biochem. 2010a;396:290–7. https://doi.org/10.1016/j.ab.2009.09.009.
26. Lao Y, Xing D, Yang S, Xiang L. Noninvasive photoacoustic imaging of the developing vasculature during early tumor growth. Phys Med Biol. 2008;53:4203–12. https://doi.org/10.1088/0031-9155/53/15/013.
27. Beard P. Biomedical photoacoustic imaging. Interface Focus. 2011;1:602–31.
28. Song LA, Maslov K, Shung KK, Wang LHV. Ultrasound-array-based real-time photoacoustic microscopy of human pulsatile dynamics in vivo. J Biomed Opt. 2010;15:021303.
29. Zaidi H, Ojha N, Morich M, et al. Design and performance evaluation of a whole body ingenuity TF PET-MRI system. Phys Med Biol. 2011;56:3091–106.
30. Behm CZ, Lindner JR. Cellular and molecular imaging with targeted contrast ultrasound. Ultrasound Q. 2006;22(1):67–72.
31. Paefgen V, Doleschel D, Kiessling F. Evolution of contrast agents for ultrasound imaging and ultrasound-mediated drug delivery. Front Pharmacol. 2015;6:197.
32. Kang ST, Yeh CK. Ultrasound microbubble contrast agents for diagnostic and therapeutic applications: current status and future design. Med J. 2012;35(2):125–39.
33. Kiessling F, Fokong S, Bzyl J, Lederle W, Palmowski M, Lammers T. Recent advances in molecular, multimodal and theranostic ultrasound imaging. Adv Drug Deliv Rev. 2014;72:15–27.
34. Wang S, Mauldin FW Jr, Klibanov AL, Hossack JA. Ultrasound-based measurement of molecular marker concentration in large blood vessels: a feasibility study. Ultrasound Med Biol. 2015;41(1):222–34.
35. Kedziorek DA, Kraitchman DL. Super-paramagnetic iron oxide labeling of stem cells for MRI tracking and delivery in cardiovascular disease. Methods Mol Biol. 2010;660:171–83. https://doi.org/10.1007/978-1-60761-705-1-11.
36. Arbab AS, Wilson LB, Ashari P, Jordan EK, Lewis BK, Frank JA. A model of lysosomal metabolism of dextran coated super-paramagnetic iron oxide (SPIO) nanoparticles: implications for cellular magnetic resonance imaging. NMR Biomed. 2005;18(6):383–9.
37. Borny R, Lechleitner T, Schmiedinger T, et al. Nucleophilic cross-linked, dextran coated iron oxide nanoparticles as basis for molecular imaging: synthesis, characterization, visualization and comparison with previous product. Contrast Media Mol Imaging. 2015;10(1):18–27.
38. Gold DV, Modrak DE, Ying Z, Cardillo TM, Sharkey RM, Goldenberg DM. New MUC1 serum immunoassay differentiates pancreatic cancer from pancreatitis. J Clin Oncol. 2006;24(2):252–8.
39. Xue S, Wang Y, Wang M, et al. Iodinated oil-loaded, fluorescent mesoporous silica-coated iron oxide nanoparticles for magnetic resonance imaging/computed tomography/fluorescence trimodal imaging. Int J Nanomedicine. 2014;9(1):2527–38.
40. Bogdanov A Jr, Matuszewski L, Bremer C, et al. Oligomerization of paramagnetic substrates result in signal amplification and can be used for MR imaging of molecular targets. Mol Imaging. 2002;1(1):16–23.
41. Qin LC, Zhao X, Hirahara K, Miyamoto Y, Ando Y, Iijima S. The smallest cardon nanotube. Nature. 2000;408(6808):50.
42. Power S, Slattery MM, Lee MJ. Nanotechnology and its relationship to interventional radiology. Part I: imaging. Cardiovasc Intervent Radiol. 2011;34(2):221–6.
43. Thrall JH. Nanotechnology and medicine. Radiology. 2004;230(2):315–8.
44. Harisinghani M. Nanoparticle-enhanced MRI: are we there yet? Lancet Oncol. 2008;9(9):814–5.

45. Coto-García AM, Sotelo-González E, Fernández-Argüelles MT, Pereiro R, Costa-Fernández JM, Sanz-Medel A. Nanoparticles as fluorescent labels for optical imaging and sensing in genomics and proteomics. Anal Bioanal Chem. 2011;399(1):29–42.
46. Kalambur VS, Longmire EK, Bischof JC. Cellular level loading and heating of superparamagnetic iron oxide nanoparticles. Langmuir. 2007;23(24):12329–36.
47. Yang X, Stein EW, Ashkenazi S, Wang LV. Nanoparticles for photoacoustic imaging. Wiley Interdiscip Rev Nanomed Nanobiotechnol. 2009;1(4):360e8.
48. Thakur ML. Genomic biomarkers for molecular imaging. Semin Nucl Med. 2009;39:236–49.
49. Aboagye EO, Kraeber-Bodéré F. Highlights lecture EANM 2016: "Embracing molecular imaging and multi-modal imaging: a smart move for nuclear medicine towards personalized medicine". Eur J Nucl Med Mol Imaging. 2017;44:1559–74.

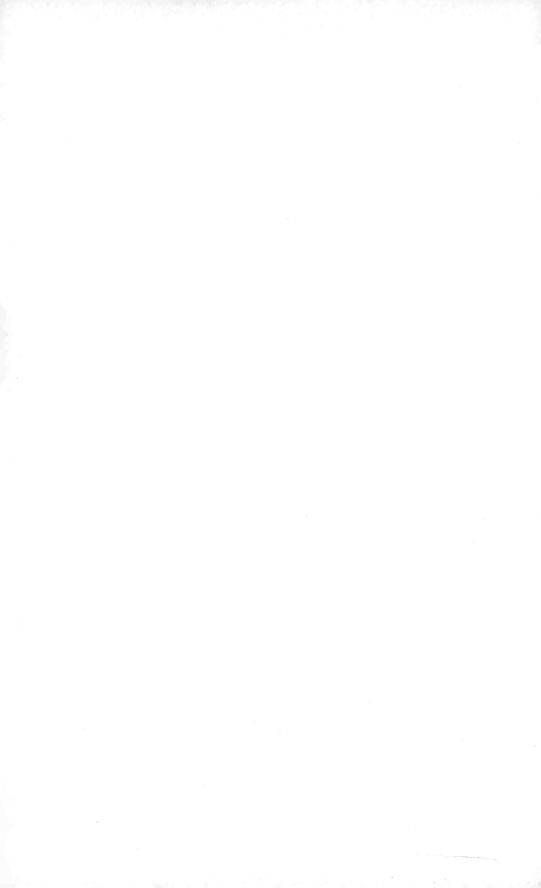